The Joshua Diet

GARY TEMPLE BODLEY

Other Titles by Gary Temple Bodley

The Teachings of Joshua

A Perception of Reality

Health, Wealth, & Love

A Radical Change
in your approach to life

Visit

THETEACHINGSOFJOSHUA.COM

Dedication

I cannot imagine life without my wife Lili who I love and adore. I see now how the Law of Attraction worked to bring us together. The way in which we came together was magical and it set the stage for our love to grow and blossom. I can't imagine another couple so perfectly matched, but I realize that when you allow what you want to manifest, perfection is the most likely result.

As we now enter nearly twenty years together and another three years with Joshua, our love continues to grow and evolve. Joshua has brought a whole new quality to this relationship as you might imagine and we are blessed to be a part of this incredible process of conscious awakening and co-creation.

Contents

Acknowledgments

I am blessed to have so many supportive friends and teachers. Again, I'd like to show my love and appreciation for Debra Jo Bright who was with us right from the beginning. Debra Jo is responsible for all of the amazing Joshua Art Quotes which can be seen on the website and received in the weekly newsletters.

I would also like to acknowledge Samantha Curtis for all the support and work she has done to spread Joshua's message. We don't know where all of this is going, but we're having fun along the way.

Steve Fanizza and Kyla Hinton, members of the Joshua Roundtable and Joshua Live podcasts, continue to give of their time and of themselves in order to broadcast the energy of Joshua's message. We have so much fun together, but I want them to know how much they mean to me.

Thanks to Jewels Johnson, Joshua not only writes through me, but is now speaking through me as well. It was Jewels who foresaw this evolution even when I was a bit skeptical. She is a trained hypnotist and while under her suggestion, Joshua emerged channeled through my voice for the very first time. Jewels has said the Joshua is the expansion of the law of attraction and with her help Joshua has now expanded their channels of communication.

I would also like to thank all of the wonderful people who contributed to the design and production of this book. From all of the proofreaders to the editor, from the production designer to the cover artist; thank you all.

And most of all, I owe all of this to Esther Hicks and the Teachings of Abraham!

My Story

It has been three years since Joshua abruptly entered my life and boy how things have changed. There was no way to see this coming and if you were to tell me this story a decade ago, I would have said you were crazy. In just three years, four books have been written, hundreds of questions have been answered, and dozens of articles and podcasts have been sent out over the airwaves. I have found a new passion and purpose in life and have gathered many truly wonderful friends along the way. What a ride!

I have always had a bit of struggle with my weight. I have a naturally lean body and it feels unpleasant to carry around an extra thirty pounds. I don't consider myself fat, but I certainly don't feel as good as I should in my body. For years I have been trying and trying to lose wight. I have tried lots of diets and programs as well as continuous exercise, but nothing ever works for very long. I was just about to give up when I asked Joshua one simple question: "Why don't diets work?" That question inspired them to write this book.

Like the three previous books, one day I wake up and Joshua says, "Write, write, write," and I get up and start typing away at my computer. I never know what I am writing when it first starts, I just receive the thoughts and put them into words. It takes about an hour a day typing furiously and each day produces three or four pages. The words are never edited, I only fix typos. In eight weeks, a book is completed.

There are no outlines, no plans, and no research, it's all just ideas and thoughts translated into words. You cannot tell where I stopped writing one day and where I picked up the next. It's very fluid. I start where I left off not even rereading the previous day's words. It's exactly as if I am typing out a fully completed book that was there before I started.

There is a reason diets don't work. It has nothing to do with food, exercise, genes, fat, calories, sugar, or any of that. It all has to do with you. Once you get that, you will discover how to alter your life in such a way that weight is no longer an issue. You will attract the lean body you desire. The side effect of reading this book will be an understanding of how you can attract anything you want, not just a healthy body. You will know how to attract financial abundance, wonderful relationships, increased joy, and everything else you want. If you can create the body you desire, then you can create the life you desire as well. It's the exact same process.

If you are not already aware, Joshua is a group of nonphysical teachers who have come to share their knowledge of the laws of the universe and the mechanism of physical reality. They see our lives and our planet from a much higher and broader perspective. They have access to infinite intelligence. They know how the system works.

From this point on, every word you will read comes straight from Joshua.

Overview

Diets don't work for most people. Will power is not sustainable for most people. When we say most people, we mean 99 percent. The only way to manifest the slim, strong and lean body you want is by first achieving a healthy and fit mind. You see, your mind controls your body, but you act as if your mind is a slave to the whims, pangs, complaints, pains, and desires emanating from your body. This is not the case. You simply have not practiced strengthening your mind.

If your body sends signals to the mind and the mind cannot or will not deal with the signals, your body will ask you to do things that are not in your best interest. Your body wants to feel good. It wants to eat, it wants to sleep, it wants to rest, and it wants to slow down. Don't let it. Don't succumb to the whims and whines of your body. Your mind controls your body. A healthy mind will be able to overcome the requests of the body.

In this book you will learn how the mind controls the body, how your emotional state of being affects the body, how your beliefs contribute to the body's function and form, how your feelings about your body impact your own goals, and how to accept your body as it is before asking it to be something different.

We are asking you to completely shift your perspective about the subject of weight, fat, eating, exercising, and diets in general. You know diets do not work for you. You know something has to change. You know you lack the ability to control your weight. You have been asking for something radically different that will really be effective. This book will describe a new approach to weight loss that is effective and that will work. It is not based on calories, or scales, or exercise, or positive thinking, or tracking movement, or keeping a food log, or cutting carbs, or sugar, or gluten, or any of that.

There is one way to maintain your body and one way only; through the power of your mind. Until you've trained your mind how to think, you cannot expect the long-term results you desire. It all has to do with the thoughts that enter your head and how you choose to deal with them.

This book utilizes infinite intelligence and the powers of the universe to leverage information in a way that is transformative. There is nothing you need to do to create the body you desire other than to build the most important muscle in your body: your brain.

Introduction

There is a way to maintain perfect health and a body that feels good to you. It has nothing to do with the food you eat, what you weigh, calories, fat, exercise, or any of that. The way to a healthy body is through the mind. A fit body is the result of a healthy, happy, focused mind.

This may seem counter-intuitive. You think that if you want to lose weight, you must simply eat less fattening foods and exercise more. It's a simple fact that if you reduce caloric intake and increase caloric burn, you'll lose all that fat and return to a perfectly lean body. If this was the case, then anyone who ever started a diet would easily and effortlessly lose the weight. Yet, it is perfectly clear to everyone reading this book that it just doesn't work like that.

Your body is made up of energy and to a large extent is formed by the thoughts you think and the beliefs you hold onto. Many of your beliefs are extremely beneficial, and for the most part you are living the life you intended to live. Generally, you consider your life to be good, but when it comes to your weight, something is stuck. No matter how hard you try, you just can't seem to lose weight and keep it off. Have you ever asked yourself why?

In the past, when you've lost weight and felt good, what happened? Were you able to keep the weight off or did it come right back? It usually comes back and there's a very good reason for that. You temporarily change your mind, which allows you to alter your attitude and approach to life. As you change your vibration, you create an environment in which you allow yourself to receive inspiration. This inspiration is crucial to losing weight. You must feel inspired. You must act in accordance with that inspiration. As you raise your vibration, allow inspiration to come, and adjust your attitude, you attract thoughts, feelings, beliefs, and actions that align with what is wanted. In this case, it's to lose weight.

This is exactly how you manifest everything you want. This is how you get things done. But unless you can maintain that attitude and approach to life, you'll revert back to your old habit of thought. As soon as you go back to your old approach to life, you lower your vibration, you start attracting those same limiting thoughts, and the old habits return. You are now inspired to eat the ice cream and watch your TV rather than take a walk after dinner.

Introduction

The mind attracts thoughts that resonate with the vibration you are emitting. If you are in a low emotional state, such as boredom, sadness, loneliness, depression, stress, frustration, worry, etc., the mind finds thoughts that will attempt to make you feel better. In these low emotional states of being, you attract thoughts and receive inspired action that causes you to take some action in order to feel better. What actions are you inspired to take? How about a glass of wine, a cigarette, some gossip, or maybe a slice of cheesecake?

It's not that all overweight people are experiencing negative emotion; it's that all people experience negative emotion from time to time. Some choose to argue, fight back, run, watch a movie, or remove themselves from the situation. Some choose to imbibe in food or drink. And a few are able to analyze the negative emotion, find the limiting belief, identify the fear behind the belief, prove to themselves that the fear is false, and adopt a perspective that allows them to regain their balance and feel good again.

When you learn to maintain your positive emotional state of being, you'll attract thoughts that resonate with that. You'll attract more thoughts of health and vitality, since this is what you want. The thought of eating fudge brownies will not come up for you because it does not resonate with your desire to feel good. You will not think that unhealthy food will make you feel better when you're already feeling good.

From our perspective, the obvious way to create and maintain a lean and fit body is to create an environment where you feel good most of the time. The better you feel in any given moment, the less likely you'll receive inspiration to take action that is out of alignment with what you truly desire. In order to have a lean body, you must have a healthy and focused mind. You must understand the laws of the universe and the mechanism of physical reality. To play this game, you must know the rules.

We assure you that you have the ability to completely transform your body from where it is now to where you would like it to be. There is a path to take. There is no rush; you have plenty of time. It is not necessary to go quickly. In fact, if you move too fast in the early stages, you'll have a hard time keeping up. This is a gradual process that will literally take a lifetime to master. There is no end to this journey. It is not a diet; you can eat whatever you like, but you must play by the rules. We intend to teach you what we know and help you along the way. We will give you some tools to work with and offer our guidance, but in order for you to change, you must change who you are being now, how you are approaching your life now, and how you feel about yourself now. The only thing you need to change is everything. As a result, your weight will change, and so will your entire experience of life.

If you loved yourself, if you felt confident and worthy, if you were secure, if you approached life from a stance that everything is right as it is, if you were non-resistant, you would be free from all stress and you would maintain a weight that is ideal for your body. One important thing to remember is that you are unique and that you chose your body. The body you chose has certain unique characteristics. It is a body that was specifically designed for you and for no one else.

In its natural, healthy state, it may take a shape that's pleasing to you, or you may judge it harshly. When you compare yourself to another and you think that their body is better than yours, you deny yourself the power and the recognition that you chose your body specifically to enable the discovery of what you're here on Earth to explore. You intended to come here to sift through life and to experience certain aspects of physical reality. You chose your specific body — its size, shape, color, and all of its qualities — as part of the trajectory that would lead you to the experiences in this life that you intended to explore.

If you have issues with your body, it's due to your habit of comparison. We will teach you to compare how you feel now to how you felt before. You will learn to compare you to you, not to anyone else. If you feel good in your body because it's naturally healthy and attractive, you will own all the power that comes with your body. If you condemn your body or yourself because you think it should be different, you cause inner conflict and stress on the body and you won't feel good.

You are starting at this point in time. You have a body that you believe is not in its ideal shape or condition. You seek improvement. You have birthed a desire to create a good-feeling, healthy, and lean body. However, you believe the way to the body you prefer is by shedding the body you have now. This is a flawed premise. The only way to a better body is to love the body you have exactly as it is. You cannot move to any improved condition by hating the present condition. You cannot change your body by thinking there is something wrong with it. You get what you are focused on. You move into a state of allowing by accepting that what exists now is perfect as it is.

You may fear that if you begin to love your body as it is now, you will never get the body you want. The laws of the universe say the opposite is true. If you can accept your present conditions, you can create future conditions that reflect your preferences. If you condemn the present conditions, your focus on them will cause them to become even more unpleasant. You get what you focus on. You get what you think about. Fighting against what you do not like brings more of it into your experience. Trusting that everything is right as it is in this moment moves you into a state of being where you can allow everything you want to flow to you. This is universal law. It works every single time, with no exceptions. We will teach you how to operate within these laws.

Chapter One

The Starting Point

You came to this environment we call physical reality for the tangible experience of it. Prior to your birth, you set certain intentions for this life. You intended to experience joy, freedom, happiness, perfect health, a lean body, and many other wonderful things this world has to offer. You also intended to explore certain specific aspects of physical reality. These are your interests and your passions.

In order to fulfill your intentions, you needed to launch yourself on a trajectory that would lead you in the direction of your interests and passions. To do so, you chose your parents and the time and place of your birth. You also chose the characteristics of your body. All of these choices you made created the conditions of your youth, and you knew these conditions would spark certain desires that would lead you to your passions.

If you did not have the parents you had, you might live a completely different life. If you were not born at the exact time and place of your birth, you might lead a completely different life. If your body was different than it is, you would certainly have led a different life. You have a life that is the result of your desires and predominance of thought, which includes your beliefs. Your life is the reflection of your vibration. What is in your life now perfectly matches your vibration. Most of it is very, very good, but there are some things you may wish to change. In order for these things to change, your vibration must change first.

Where you are is the perfect place to start. The life you have led has caused you to birth certain desires, and from that you are choosing to approach life in a certain manner. Your habit is to fix what's broken. If something doesn't work, you toss it out and get a new one. But you can't fix your body because your body is the perfect representation of your vibration. In other words, you created the body you see in the mirror, down to the tiniest detail.

You are the creator of you and you can create whatever you like. You have the ability to be, do, and have everything you want in this reality. The universe yields to your wishes as long as you understand how your point of focus creates your reality. Since you created your body, you must not dislike it. It is the creation you chose, even though your choices were made unconsciously. In this book we hope to show you how to make conscious choices that will mold your body (and your entire life) in a way that you prefer.

Where you are now is perfect. Your body is perfect. You are perfect. The conditions of your life are perfect. The conditions in this very moment are perfect. Everything is right just the way it is. There is nothing wrong with any of it. The perception you are choosing causes you to believe it is wrong, but you are choosing to look at it from a narrow, limited perspective. From the higher perspective, everything is right. When you believe that something is wrong, you hold onto that, and you are not able to change. When you focus on what's wrong, your vibration emits it out to the universe, and the universe brings more of that into your life. Everything comes back to you by the thoughts you think, the words you speak, and the actions you take, all of which are out of alignment with what you want.

When you feel fat, you attract thoughts, words, and actions that reinforce how you feel. You are meant to feel good, and the universe was designed to reinforce your good feelings with kind words, nice thoughts, and beneficial actions. When you feel bad, whether it is feeling fat, feeling lonely, feeling bored, feeling trapped, feeling frustrated, etc., the universe responds with thoughts that match how you feel. You then continue this by speaking words that describe your unwanted feelings. You receive inspiration to act in a way that causes you to continue feeling the way you do. It is all caused by the way you feel. How you feel creates your vibration, which emits a signal, and the universe responds to that signal. It's called the Law of Attraction.

Have you ever been angry and received the thought that you should hit the person who made you angry? You might not have physically hit the person, but you might have attacked them verbally. You felt bad, and the universe sent you thoughts to try to make you feel better. Feeling anger is a low-vibrational feeling, and that vibration attracts similar low-vibrational thoughts. The thoughts feel like inspiration to act, because from that low-emotional state of being, that's all you have access to.

Thoughts come to you based on the vibration you're emitting. If you're having fun, fun thoughts come. If you're feeling depressed, depressing thoughts come. The thoughts are a match to the vibration. If you feel fat, you will attract thoughts that make you feel bad, because even though the thoughts are a match to your vibration, they are out of alignment with who you really are and what you really want. That's why they feel bad. Your negative emotion is your indication that the perspective you are choosing is not aligned with your highest good.

II.

You are on the right path. Something you are doing, or wanting, or feeling has already caused a shift in your vibration and you are attracting what you want. It is coming to you, and you are allowing it to come. The evidence is right there in front of you. If you have somehow found this book, you attracted it into your life. You have managed to become a vibrational match to the ideas found in this book.

This is how attraction works. You birth a desire, and the universe responds to your desire. As soon as you want something, the universe is on the job. It's bringing it to you. You just have to be open to it when it comes. You have to allow it to come to you. If you resist it, it cannot come.

Somehow, you found this book, and that means your vibration is a match to it. You are also a match to us. Your vibration has led you here, and that means you are meant to be here. This book is beneficial. It's for your higher good. Maybe you were given the book by a friend. If you accepted the book and managed to read this far into it, you have allowed it to come into your reality. That is a very good thing indeed. Many, many people will be led to this book. Some will allow it to enter their reality and some will not. Those who resist it have a limiting belief, and that belief is based in some irrational fear. They may have thoughts like, "This sounds too good to be true. This won't work for me. I don't believe that the mind has anything to do with the body. I don't believe that a group of nonphysical teachers exists,." That is all just resistance. If something comes to you, it is a match to your vibration. If it resonates with you on any level, it's worth exploring further.

What you have lived up to this point has brought you here. Where you are now is the perfect place to start. Forget about the past. The past led you to this moment in time. That is a very good thing. Forget about the future. What you do in this moment dictates how that future will unfold.

You have a choice to make. You can believe that everything wrong happened and that's how you ended up here, or you can believe that everything happened perfectly so that you could be here now. The choice you make will have a lot to do with how your future unfolds from this point forward. Realize that everything is right, that everything is okay, that your past experience created desires and those desires led you here. You're already this far in. You found us. You found this book. That is proof that everything is right. That is proof that your vibration is leading you right where you want to go. That is proof that you're willing and able to make a change. Good for you!

III.

You have a desire to create a lean body. You believe that by having a lean body, you'll feel better. Maybe you will and maybe you won't. The reason you want anything in life is because you think it will make you feel better. However, you really don't know for sure if that's true. Sometimes you get what you think you want and realize that you don't feel any better after all. This has to do with feelings of worthiness.

You are worthy of living the life you desire. You are a worthy being, as worthy as any who has ever lived. There is not another person on Earth who is more worthy than you. There is not another who is less worthy either. You came to this physical world to explore things that interest you. You have just as much right to do that as anyone. However, when you choose to compare your life or yourself to anyone else, you may wish for things to be different. You might assume their lives are better because they, as people, are better. That's just not the case.

By comparing yourself to someone else, you are seeing the surface or the facade of that person. You cannot know if they are happy or not. You cannot know what their struggles are. You cannot know if they feel as worthy as you or anyone else. You just see the shiny exterior, but you cannot know what lies beneath. So it is time to stop comparing yourself to others and realize that you are just as worthy as anyone else.

Think of Earth as an amusement park, like Disneyland. You came here because you thought it would be fun and exhilarating. You go to Disneyland because you think it will be fun and exhilarating. When you buy your ticket and enter through the gates, you don't believe that you are better or worse than any other fun-seeker there. You believe you have just as much right to ride any ride and see any attraction as the next person. There's no plausible reason to believe you are any less worthy than anyone else on this playground called Earth. You've paid your ticket and you are here. That means you are worthy to be here.

You are worthy enough to live the life you desire. You are worthy enough to love and to be loved. You are worthy enough to have the body you desire. But don't for a moment believe that having a nice body will make you feel worthy. It will not.

If you want something because you think it will make you feel better about yourself, it won't. If you think having a lean body, being attractive, having money, having an attractive mate, having fame, or having anything else will make you feel worthy, it simply will not. You see, the universe does not work in reverse. You must feel good first, and the universe will respond to how you feel. If you feel fat (bad), getting lean won't make you feel thin (good). You'll still feel fat, because being leaner won't change anything. If you don't feel worthy, your life won't change just because you're a little thinner. If you don't feel worthy, your life won't change by getting plastic surgery. If you don't feel worthy, your life won't change by making money, or getting married, or having a baby, or becoming famous. If you don't feel worthy, you'll constantly choose a limited perspective and you'll continue to feel bad. You must strive to feel good first and feel that you're already worthy, and then you'll receive thoughts and manifestations that reflect how you feel.

Feeling good is the only thing that really matters. This is a feeling reality. Have you ever thought about that? All you're ever doing in any moment is feeling. You're either feeling good, content, pleasant, happy, secure, etc., or you're feeling bad, scared, worried, insecure, bored, etc.

It doesn't matter what's happening in the outside world; you are either choosing to look at stuff that makes you feel good or at stuff that makes you feel bad. You choose what to look at, you chose the perspective, and you choose whether you feel good or bad. It's all up to you.

If you have a habit of looking at things that make you feel good, then good for you. This is how reality was designed. It was thought that you would focus on things you preferred and you would receive good feelings to reinforce your habit of looking at good-feeling stuff. If occasionally you looked at something in a way that was out of alignment with what you wanted, you would receive a little jolt in the form of negative emotion. This is a bad feeling, and it was thought that you would quickly change your perspective to see the subject in a way that would make you feel good again. You see something you don't like, so you receive negative emotion, which doesn't feel good, and you turn to a better-feeling thought or perspective. But that's not what happens, is it?

No, it's not. You receive negative emotion, and you keep looking at what you don't want. You get so used to feeling bad that it doesn't really feel that bad any more. You start to accept the negative emotion as a part of life. You believe that the conditions of the outside world cause you to feel good or bad, and you have no power over that. We're here to tell you that this was not intended. This is not part of the design. You can learn to feel good and to change your perspective when you don't feel good. You can become used to feeling good. Feeling good is the most important thing you can do to improve the quality of your experience of life. While we would never want you to lose the ability to experience negative emotion, we would like to stress the value of feeling good as much of the time as possible.

When you strive to feel good, when you intend to feel good, you set forth powerful energies out into the universe. The universe yields to how you feel. When you feel strong, confident, loving, happy, funny, exuberant, etc., the universe must bring you evidence of how you are feeling. You will encounter more fun, more love, more satisfaction, more success, and more moments that reinforce your good feelings. It is just the design of the system.

When you feel bad, the universe must alert you. If the universe did not create moments that caused you to feel bad, how would you know that your vibration was emitting a frequency that was out of alignment with who you really are or what you really want? The negative emotion is a signal to alter your focus. You're looking at something in a way that does not help you get what you want.

Feel good now and you will attract a body that also feels good. Is it a leaner body? Maybe, but who cares? If it feels good to you, then isn't that what really matters? If it is a healthy, energetic, and vibrant body, isn't that a good thing? Does it have to look like a supermodel's body for you to be happy? Certainly not. You can be happy with the body you have now and over time that body will cause you to feel happy. It's how you feel about the body that matters most.

Chapter Two

Emotional Triggers and Set Points

There are two types of fear: rational and irrational. Rational fear is part of the survival instinct, and it keeps you alive and out of harm's way. You are supposed to feel fear in the presence of real danger. Anything that can kill you or cause injury initiates a rational fear. When you are hiking in the woods and you encounter a bear, rational fear is a useful thing. Otherwise, you might want to walk up to the bear and give him a cuddle.

Irrational fear comes up when you encounter something scary but that cannot kill or physically harm you. It is irrational to fear public speaking or asking someone for a date. It is irrational fear that stops you from doing a lot of things you would like to do. Irrational fear is limiting.

When you birth a desire, the universe goes to work to manifest that desire into your reality. In order for this to happen, you must change. You see, the version of you that exists right now is represented by your vibration. Everything you have in your life right now, including your physical body, is a match to your vibration. If it exists in your life, it is a match to you. If it does not exist, you are not yet a match to it. In order to become a vibrational match to anything you do not have, you must change your vibration. Your vibration is made up of the thoughts you think, the beliefs you hold, your inner feelings, and your approach to life. In order to change your vibration to get what you want, you must change those things.

You actually do not have to do anything at all other than allow the change to take place. The universe will make the changes to you that will modify your vibration if you allow it. The universe will put you in certain situations that will cause you to rethink your beliefs. If you go along with it by allowing the changes to occur, your desire will manifest into your reality. However, if you resist these manifestation events, you will not change and your desire cannot manifest.

There is something in your belief system that is causing you to hold onto unwanted weight. It could be anything, so there's no reason to try to identify it. The universe knows what it is and it will help you if you allow it. The universe will place you in certain situations called Manifestation Events, that will cause you to feel emotion both positive and negative. When something happens and you feel positive emotion, such as joy, love, appreciation, laughter, excitement, exhilaration, etc., this is a manifestation event that is alerting you to some very beneficial beliefs. Whatever the subject is, you are looking at it in a way that fully aligns with your desire, and this will allow your desire to manifest.

When you feel negative emotion, such as hatred, anger, jealousy, rage, loneliness, boredom, apathy, etc., this is an indication that you are looking at the subject in a way that goes against everything you want. Whenever you feel bad, it means your perspective on the subject is off. You're off track. You're moving away from what you want. You have some limiting belief about the subject and this belief is based in irrational fear.

If the fear is irrational, meaning it can't kill you, then it is false. All irrational fears are false. They seem real, but they are not. You can prove that an irrational fear is false. You can find evidence that it is false. When you show yourself evidence that the irrational fear is false, you reduce the intensity of that fear. As soon as you do, you'll feel relief. When you feel relief, it is an indication that you've reduced the intensity of the fear and you've altered your perspective to one that supports what you want. You're back on track.

It may take a little practice to start realizing that every time you feel negative emotion you're in the middle of a manifestation event. Because you feel sad, angry, upset, or whatever, you will feel that the situation is wrong. You will want to justify your emotions by making yourself right and the thing wrong. But the only reason you're feeling bad is because you're feeling fear. It is not that the thing is wrong; it's just that there is some fear making you believe it's wrong or bad. Find the fear, prove it's false, and you'll reduce the intensity of the fear.

Do you know what happens when you reduce the intensity of fear? You increase the intensity and capacity for love and you raise your vibration. By altering the fear, you modify your vibration. As your vibration changes, so does your world. Your reality is simply a reflection of your vibration. Every time your vibration raises, your world gets a little bigger and brighter.

Whenever you feel negative emotion, stop and think about it. Why do you feel bad? What's the limiting belief? What's the irrational fear at the base of this limiting belief? What evidence can you find to prove it's false? Now that you've proven the fear is false, do you feel better? If so, you reduced the intensity of that fear and you've raised your vibration.

Manifestation events occur several times per day. Soon you will start thinking about them as they occur. At first it may take a few hours or days to realize you were in one. That doesn't matter. If you can analyze the event and feel better as a result, you've done the necessary work. As you practice this, you'll get better at finding the fear. You'll also get quicker. You'll soon form a habit and as these events come up, you'll squash the fears left, right, and center.

II.

The basis of this earthly environment is well-being. You are meant to feel good. Your natural emotional state of being is ease. Without the contrast that comes into your life, you would feel good all the time. However, you came here to expand, and you expand as a result of contrast. Things happen and from those events you create preferences. You are here to create your reality, experience life, and move toward your preferences. In the process, you feel good sometimes and bad other times.

When you feel good, you have access to good-feeling thoughts. When you feel bad, you have access to low-vibrational thoughts, many of which are there to improve how you feel. They are quick fixes. They bring only temporary satisfaction. Some of these thoughts inspire you to action, which results in your feeling even worse. In order to gain the control you desire, you must understand how the system works. You're unable to lose the weight you want and to bring into reality the lean body you want because your thoughts are sabotaging your success. You have no control over your own thoughts and this is the root of the issue.

The thoughts you think are not manufactured in your head. Did you know that? All thoughts exist in the nonphysical, and your vibration attracts the thoughts that resonate with how you're feeling in the moment. Thoughts are the first manifestation created by your vibrational signal. You emit a vibration and you attract things into your reality. The first things you attract are thoughts. Keep the momentum going and the thoughts turn into physical conditions. They can be physical objects or physical experiences. These physical things are a match to your vibration. They are a match to how you are feeling.

Change the way you feel and you change what the universe brings to you. Change your emotional state of being and you change the quality of thoughts that come to you. When you feel good, you attract thoughts that match how you feel. When you feel bad, you attract similar low-vibrational thoughts. Thoughts create inspiration to act. You might be inspired to say something or do something. The type of things you say and do stem from your emotional state of being. When you are flying high emotionally, you say and do things with love. When you are in a low-emotional state of being, you say and do things out of fear.

When you feel good, you are moving along a path toward what is wanted. If you want it and you feel good, you are allowing it to come to you. When you feel bad, you are more likely to focus on the negative aspects of the conditions around you, and that will keep you bound to the things you do not prefer. When you feel good, you feel like you're moving along and making progress. When you feel bad, you feel like you're stuck in a rut.

By now we hope you can see the importance of feeling good. The reason you cannot lose the weight and create the good-feeling body you want is because you don't feel good enough of the time to offset the sabotage that is done during the times you don't feel good. You may feel good 90 percent of the time, and during these times you eat right and do everything that makes sense to achieve your goal of losing weight. However, during the times you feel bad, you reach for something that offsets the gains you've made. It has nothing to do with your physical body; it has to do with the thoughts you attract during those times when you don't feel good.

Unless you understand this aspect of the system, you cannot know how to accomplish any goal. When you understand that certain qualities of thought are attracted based on your emotional state of being, you can set intentions for what is wanted, and this will help you work within the system itself rather than trying to fight the system. Unless you understand that your entire mission is ruined by short durations of sabotage, you can't solve the problem. So here it is:

Physical reality is a place you chose to enter to experience life, expand through experience, and encounter contrast so that you could define preferences.

This is a system that has certain laws and principles, and if you want to achieve your goals, you must learn the laws and how the mechanism of physical reality works.

You don't create thoughts; you attract thoughts. Every thought you think is being attracted based on your emotional state of being. When you feel good, you have access to good-feeling and empowering thoughts. When you allow yourself to feel bad, you have a more limited access to thoughts, and most of the thoughts available to you are based in fear.

When you feel good, you'll receive inspiration to act, which will move you along your path to what it is you want. If you want to create a lean, healthy body, you will be inspired to eat certain foods and do certain things that will move you in the direction of what is wanted.

When you feel bad, you will be inspired to act in a way that will temporarily relieve or adjust how you feel. You will receive inspiration to do things that cause temporary relief but set you back in terms of reaching the manifestation of your desire.

Think about how you feel and realize that the thoughts coming to you are there because of the way you're feeling in the moment. Adjust how you feel and you will attract better-feeling thoughts. You can control how you feel in every moment by consciously choosing better-feeling thoughts. When you don't feel good and you simply allow thoughts to flow to you, those thoughts will resonate with your vibrational tone. However, when you're conscious of what's really happening, you can reach for better-feeling thoughts. By doing this, you alter your vibration on your own. You make the effort and are rewarded with thoughts that match a higher vibration. Those thoughts build momentum and soon you are out of the negative emotional state and back to feeling good again.

III.

When you were born, your natural emotional set point was very high. When you felt bad, you really noticed it, and you cried and screamed. Even if you felt just a little bad, you made enough noise to wake the entire house. You felt very good most of the time and when you felt bad, you did not stand for it. This is how you were designed.

Over time you got used to feeling bad and now feeling bad is a normal part of everyday life. You are numb to your feelings. You believe it is normal to sometimes feel good and sometimes feel bad, but that is not normal. You believe it is normal to suppress your emotions, but it is not normal. You are meant to feel good almost all the time and when you feel bad you are meant to understand what is happening and to get back to feeling good quickly. You are not meant to reach for something external to make yourself feel good again. You are meant to feel good by reaching for better-feeling thoughts until you feel relief.

By not understanding how the system works, you automatically reach for some external substance or action to bring you satisfaction and relief. This is fine as long as you know what you're really doing. When you feel low energy and reach for a caffeinated beverage, you will receive a temporary jolt of energy. However, this is a quick fix and has ramifications that might offset the strides you've made toward your goal. If you're feeling bored, you might reach for a sweet treat. This is fine as long as you are consciously aware of what you're doing. However, it's the habit of reaching for something external that causes you to veer off your path. When you look for a fix outside yourself, you cause a shift in the way you find relief from internal to external. This habit can be traced back to your infancy and childhood.

There is momentum created in every aspect of physical reality. When you start doing anything, good or bad, you create a certain amount of thrust behind it. If you were to start walking every day, pretty soon your body would feel the need to walk. If you were to start smoking every day, pretty soon your body would feel the need to smoke. When you start reaching for external methods to move you to a different state of being, you will form a habit, which is another term for expressing the word "momentum." Habit is momentum and momentum is habit. Looking for external methods to adjust your emotional state of being is your habit and this habit has a lot of momentum behind it. Your habit was created as a result of this physical experience. It is a habit formed at birth and it is not your fault.

When you were born, you felt hunger and you sought relief by crying, and soon you were given food. When you felt alone, you cried, and soon you were soothed in the arms of your mother. When you felt pain, you were cared for by someone outside you. When you were a child and you were bored, you looked for things in this physical world to distract you and you moved from one state of being to another. This is a physical reality, and there are so many things outside of you that will help you change your emotional state. You cannot be blamed for adopting this habit. It is simply part of life.

But you must also realize that you have access to conscious awareness at all times. If you can maintain your focus on how you feel, you can adjust your emotional state at any time simply by being aware of those times when you feel a dip, realizing that your tendency will be to reach for outside fixes, realizing that the thoughts that are flowing to you have been attracted by your state of being, and understanding that you have the ability to reach for better-feeling thoughts. This is how you slowly overcome your longest-held and most powerful habits.

IV.

All humans have certain fears and when those fears are triggered by an outside event or influence, their emotional state of being quickly drops. You could be in the middle of a fun time relaxing with your mate when he or she says something that offends you without even knowing it. Your fear is triggered in that moment and you react to the comment by moving into a low vibrational state of being. You might get angry, upset, sad, disappointed, or any one of a number of negative emotions.

Triggers carry with them the long tail of momentum. You've had these triggers for a very long time and when they appear, you have almost no control over your emotions. Triggers are usually set off by someone close to you. It's often a parent, sibling, or spouse. The closer you are to that person, the more powerful the trigger can be. But, like all emotions, you have the ability to understand what is happening, identify the trigger, and release its power by thinking better thoughts. You can always maintain your emotional state of being no matter what's happening in the world around you. It just takes practice and awareness.

When emotional triggers come up, you must reach for relief. If you can soothe yourself by thinking better-feeling thoughts, then that is a wonderful thing. If you can analyze the fear and engage the art of analysis by proving to yourself that the fear is false, that is the best way to ease the intensity of these triggers in the future. However, without realizing it, you are likely to reach for some external substance to relieve your negative emotion. It might be a cigarette, a drink, or a piece of cake. When you reach for something outside of you to soothe your emotional pain, you sabotage some of the progress made toward that which you are wanting.

Triggers are important to understand because they often come up without warning. Your response to them is predictable because it's a habit. You've responded the same way to the same triggers for a very long time. Now it's time to reduce the effect these triggers have on your emotional state of being. Triggers are so dangerous because you can't often tell when they're happening. Your fear in this area is so strong and you feel like you have no control over your reactions. The worse part is that you may be happy and engaged all day long and one offhand comment can send you reeling backwards. The beneficial momentum you create by being focused the entire day can be undone by a reaction to a trigger. It doesn't seem fair.

The fact is that you have not been aware of the effects of triggers. You have done nothing to prepare yourself. You haven't done the work to remove the intensity of the trigger. Actually, it's really quite simple when you take the time to analyze any trigger. You can overcome the negative effect of triggers by first being aware that they exist and being prepared for them when they come.

Most of the time when something seemingly bad happens, you can see it coming. Usually when you are in a high-vibrational state of being, you can maintain your good mood and things generally go well for you as a result. When you are in a low-vibrational state of being, you have experience with the negative manifestations that occur while in that state. You understand that low-emotional states of being are likely to create manifestations that match it and you are not surprised when they come. In the case of triggers, which seem to suddenly appear out of nowhere, you are usually caught off guard and this makes the analysis process a little more challenging.

The way to deal with triggers is the same way you deal with limiting beliefs. Triggers are nothing more than highly intense limiting beliefs that have a lot of momentum behind them. Your negative reaction to a trigger tells the whole story. The way you go so quickly from feeling good to feeling bad is an indication that a powerful trigger exists. Usually it is not possible to stop in the moment the trigger is occurring and analyze it. There's just too much momentum. Typically, you will have to let the episode pass and analyze it after a duration of time has gone by. Once you've cooled down, you can look at the fear behind it and realize that like all other irrational fears, it is false.

If someone says something to you and as a result you rapidly move from a positive emotional state of being to a negative one, you've encountered a trigger. Triggers feel especially bad because the contrast between how you were feeling before the trigger and after is quite severe. But once you've regained your composure, you can look at the situation from the higher perspective and find the fear. Finding the fear here is key. Because the fear is so intense, you might have a hard time defining it. You might believe the fear is a fact of life and that it's true. But if the fear is irrational, meaning it can't kill you, then you can be assured that it's always, always false. Every single time.

By finding evidence that the fear is false, you reduce the intensity of the trigger and in the future, your reaction will be muted to a degree. The more often you practice the art of analysis, the less effect triggers will have on your emotional state of being. By reducing their effects, you maintain the momentum toward what's wanted.

V.

You have an emotional set point right now. This set point is different for you now than it was ten years ago. It is much different now than it was when you were a small child. Your emotional set point has a lot to do with your approach to life. It is influenced by how you view your world. The higher your emotional set point, the easier life is for you. When you work to consciously raise your emotional set point, you move closer to the state of allowing and from there everything you want, including a lean body, flows easily to you.

Are you generally grumpy or happy? Are you optimistic or pessimistic? Do you normally feel good or is there often something to complain about? Do you appreciate things the way they are or are there things you'd like to change? Do you enjoy being around other people or would you prefer to be left alone? Are you courageous or frightened? Can you see the difference between higher and lower emotional set points?

The better you generally feel, the easier it is for you to allow good things to come to you. You are an allower. The worse you generally feel, the more likely you are to resist the things you want. When you believe that the conditions around you, including your weight, are okay or even good, you are in the state of allowing and can allow better conditions to evolve. When you believe that the conditions around you are wrong, including your weight, and that you must work to change the conditions, you have adopted a stance of resistance and nothing will change. There's nothing you can do to change the conditions; all you can do is change yourself.

The idea here is to consciously think good-feeling thoughts about the conditions that exist in your life so that you can raise your vibrational set point and feel good more and more of the time. Feeling bad will keep you stuck and feeling good will move you forward. The real reason you want a lean body is because you think having one will make you feel good. Feel good first and the lean body will take shape on its own. It is your resistance to what is that causes what is to grow larger. Pun intended.

When you complain about your weight, or your body's inability to lose weight, or the reasons you can't take long walks or exercise, you hold yourself apart from what you want. By complaining — speaking your mind about something you think is bad or wrong — you take powerful action that focuses your powers of creation on what you do not want. By focusing on what is not wanted — excess weight — you bring more of it into your reality. It is simply the primary law of the universe at work.

By relaxing your strong opinions and feeling a bit better about the conditions, you break your focus on what is and turn toward what could be. Can life be good? Can things improve over time? Can you be making progress? Can you change your habit of thought? Can you reduce the intensity of limiting beliefs? Yes you can!

By feeling better, you improve your access to all things wanted. By demanding to feel good, you raise your vibration and the universe must respond. By expecting good things to come to you when you increase your emotional set point, good things will come. Feeling good creates momentum. The more often you feel good, the more often you will encounter good-feeling thoughts and manifestations. Seek to feel good and the universe will yield to how you feel. It is law.

Chapter Three

How the Power of Your Beliefs Forms Your Reality

What you believe to be true, is. What you expect, comes. Your thoughts form your reality. This is how physical reality was designed. If you want to change your reality, you simply change your beliefs, expectations, and thoughts.

If you had the belief that eating ice cream does not affect your weight, it would not affect your weight. Let's analyze this a bit further, because we can sense your skepticism. If you had this belief, then ice cream could not affect your weight, because if it did and you noticed it, you could not hold this belief any longer. So, for you, you either don't eat enough ice cream to make a noticeable difference in your weight or you believe that the extra weight is attributable to some other factor. Either way, you don't believe ice cream affects your weight. This is how beliefs work.

You have a belief that you believe is the truth. You consider most of your strongly held beliefs to be fact. You are so sure that they are right that you often don't even consider evidence that could prove them false. However, as soon as you encounter evidence that proves the belief is false, that belief instantly loses its intensity. It doesn't fade completely, but its power has evaporated.

Back to the ice cream example. If you believe that ice cream does not affect your weight because that has been your experience, you might live happily with this one belief that other people would not believe. It is out of the norm for people to believe this. But for you, no evidence has been found to contradict it and so you're happy to keep entertaining it. Besides, it's not a limiting belief, so what's the problem? And we quite agree. However, if you were to experiment by eating a gallon of ice cream every day for a month, you would find evidence that either definitively supports or denies your belief. If you conducted this experiment and did not gain weight, your belief would be cemented. But if you did gain weight, the intensity of this belief would be reduced and you might rephrase your belief in the future. You might form a new belief that while excessive amounts of ice cream will cause weight gain, moderate amounts will not. This belief will hold until you conduct another experiment.

All of your beliefs can be challenged in this manner, but why would you find it beneficial to do so? Because many of your beliefs are limiting. They keep you from doing what you want to do. They keep you from getting what you want. They limit your experience and you came here knowing there are no limits to what you could be, do, or have. Limiting beliefs need not be held onto for they are based in irrational fear. You can reduce the intensity of all limiting beliefs through the art of analysis, just as we did in the example above. If a belief is based in an irrational fear, the belief is false every time, and you can find evidence to prove it's false.

Many of your beliefs are highly beneficial. When you feel good, you're looking at life in a way that aligns with your beneficial beliefs. When you laugh, feel inspiration, or experience the sensation of goosebumps, you are fully aligned in the present moment with your highly beneficial beliefs. By appreciating these good-feeling moments, you increase the power of your beneficial beliefs. Beneficial beliefs are based in love and are always true. You can find evidence that proves your beneficial beliefs are true.

Limiting beliefs are false. They are based in irrational fear and this inherently means they are not true. You can find evidence that proves they're false. When you feel negative emotion in any moment, it means you are acting in a way that aligns with your limiting beliefs. You are responding to irrational fear and in doing so you are limiting your experience of life.

Reduce the intensity of your limiting beliefs and your experience will expand, you'll raise your vibration, and your beneficial beliefs will gain more power in creating the reality you prefer. When you reduce your limiting beliefs and increase your beneficial beliefs, your reality will respond to this new vibration and things will get a lot better.

II.

You have been living with your beliefs for a long time. Your reality is created by the thoughts you think and the beliefs you're attached to. Because the Law of Attraction responds to your beliefs, whether they are beneficial or limiting, you see evidence that suggests that the beliefs are valid and in doing so your beliefs become more rigid. It's not that the beliefs are true, it's just that physical reality is created around you so that it conforms to your beliefs. Therefore, what you believe becomes your reality and in doing so your beliefs become real too. They become solidified.

This is fine when it comes to beneficial beliefs. Beliefs that fully support you and what you want are your allies. Having many beneficial beliefs is a very good thing because they help to shape your reality in a way that's pleasing to you. There is no downside to having lots of highly intense beneficial beliefs. We will say that these beliefs are based in love and are true. You would not want to find evidence that weakens the intensity of a beneficial belief.

On the other hand, limiting beliefs can be just as, if not more intense than beneficial beliefs. The more intense a limiting belief, the stronger it is and the harder it is to release. If you have a limiting belief that got its start during your childhood years, that belief has likely become quite intense. It might be so intense now that you don't even consider it to be a belief. You might think that it's just part of the fabric of life. It's unavoidable. It's just how it is. It has gained momentum and it builds upon itself every time it shows up in your life. However, if it is unwanted, if it is limiting, if you feel negative emotion when it shows itself, you know it's based in fear and therefore it's false.

What could happen in childhood that might lead to the adoption of a limiting belief? Maybe your parents got divorced and one of them moved out and left you. Maybe a parent or grandparent died while you were young and you felt abandoned. Possibly something happened in school and they attached a label to you (prodigy, bully, victim, autistic, dyslexic, stupid, slow, jock, stoner, pleaser, etc.). Lots of various limiting beliefs find their way into your consciousness at a very young age and because you adopted them when you were young, they've built up quite a bit of momentum.

You can't stop momentum in its tracks; you must slowly ease around it and chip away at it a little at a time. Imagine a cargo ship cruising along in the ocean. Someone falls overboard. The ship can't just stop and reverse course. It may take miles before the ship can slow its momentum and then gradually turn around and chart a course in the other direction. It is the same with a highly intense limiting belief that got its start when you were younger. You must slowly chip away at the belief a little at a time. Consistency and diligence are key here. You do a little work each time the limiting belief pops up. This might be every day in some cases.

Many limiting beliefs emerge several times per day. Something will remind you of some hurt from your past. You might hear a song. You might smell something, or someone might say something that triggers a memory. Every time you go back to that limiting belief, you feel bad and when you feel bad, you usually look for external sources to help you feel better. Even if it's just a little thing. You might not be crying, but you might feel a hint of sadness and that is enough for thoughts to come through that will derail all the well-intentioned habits you've accumulated. All the good work has been put asunder by one brief unfocused, unconscious moment just so you can feel a little bit better. This is when you reach for the ice cream, the cigarette, or the glass of wine.

You might be able to will your way through anything for a brief period of time. However, if you do not reduce the intensity of limiting beliefs as they occur, you will simply revert back to your old habits of thought as soon as the will power fades away. This is why will power is ineffective and diets don't last.

III.

You have the ability to choose any thought and you also have the ability to choose any belief. Beliefs are not made in stone. They are illusions. Most of your beliefs have never really been tested. You carry with you a set of beliefs based on chance encounters and what other people have told you. Since they've been with you a long, long time, they've gained momentum. You believe your beliefs are true, but most are not. Now is the time to challenge your limiting beliefs and shore up your beneficial beliefs.

Limiting beliefs are based in fear and are therefore untrue. Beneficial beliefs are based in love and are therefore true. Your reality, including the shape of your body, is formed as a result of your thoughts and beliefs. Your beliefs are simply highly structured thought forms that repeat over and over again. When the world conforms to your beliefs, as it must due to the Law of Attraction, you feel validated. However, when the world conforms to your limiting beliefs, you might notice that your beliefs feel validated, but because they're limiting, they're still false.

If you would like to change any part of your life, the way to do that is to adjust your set of beliefs. If you seek improvement, the way to improve is to challenge your limiting beliefs and support your beneficial beliefs. You cannot do away with any belief completely. All you're dong is modifying the belief by lowering or raising its intensity. The more intense a belief, the more reality conforms to it. The less intense, the less a factor it is in your reality. You must understand that there is nothing random going on here. Physical reality is a closed system designed to provide you with everything you need to explore certain aspects of yourself and to expand as a result. It must yield to you, otherwise the system would not work. Thoughts and beliefs create your reality.

If you look at another person in comparison to yourself and judge yourself to be fat, then this becomes your belief and the world conforms to that one highly intense and extremely limiting belief. Now, how will that limiting belief manifest itself in your daily life? Well, if you think you are fat compared to others, then you must be right. In order to be fat, you will be inspired to eat. You will have cravings for foods that cause you to remain fat and these cravings will be powerful. It will be unpleasant to deny them and in doing so you suffer. However, when your will power breaks and you succumb to the cravings, you will feel bad and slip into a negative emotional state of being, which cuts off your access to higher vibrational thoughts and ideas.

Feeling bad feeds on itself and momentum is created. When you feel bad, you receive thoughts that resonate with that and your feelings spiral downwards. As you can imagine, this continues until you feel bad for so long you choose to call it depression or some other label. You get numb to these feelings and now it's harder to know when you're experiencing negative emotion. You get to a place where you just feel stuck and all you have access to are thoughts that match how you feel.

You must realize that you are unique and that you came to this reality to explore Earth in your own unique way. You chose your body for this mission. It is an important part of your trajectory. You will live life a certain way because of the body you chose. You have control over the body. Some parts of the body you can actively control with your mind and other parts will only yield to the influence of your thoughts. You can command your hand to wave and your legs to walk. You can blink your eyes and breathe through your nose. You can't actively control the function of your heart, liver, stomach, other organs, or the individual cells in your body, but you can and do influence all of them with your thoughts.

If you do not like certain aspects of your own body, that dislike influences your cells. If you love certain aspects of your body, this love also influences your cells. The cells of your body are influenced by how you feel and what you're thinking about. Your mind and body are inseparably linked.

You are not your body and your body is not you; however, you and your body are in this together, exploring reality. The cells of your body came here to explore life in physical reality, just as you did. Each cell in your body is an individual and unique life form living life from its own unique perspective. All cells are seeking and finding well-being. That is their natural state. All cells seek to feel good. When you feel bad, you influence your cells, which naturally want and are designed to feel good. You upset (to a degree) the well-being of your cells when you feel bad. When you feel good, you are in complete harmony with every cell in your body.

Fat cells want to feel good too. Fat cells have a reason for being. Fat cells would like to continue to provide benefit for the body. Fat cells want to be useful. Fat cells want to be burned as fuel. Fat is extremely good as a form of energy storage. Burn the fat and you'll feel good because your body will be working as it should. Hate the fat and you cause the body to behave in contrast to how it was designed.

Your body is a highly intelligent and sensitive colony of cells all working together to move you through this physical reality in this physical environment. Your cells are thrilled to be here. Together, your cells live and die and are reborn to carry you for many, many years on Earth. While your cells come and go, you are able to carry on your stream of consciousness until you decide to return to the nonphysical. In this reality, thanks in part to every cell in your body, you can be, do, and have anything you choose. Since you choose it all, why not choose to appreciate all aspects of the body you have now? By focusing your attention on one small part of the body that displeases you, you influence the entire system in a way that does not serve you or them.

When you exercise, you do not do it to rid the body of its ugly fat cells; you do it so that the body can perform its functions as it was designed to. When you eat healthy foods, you do not eat them in order to rid the body of its ugly fat; you eat these foods because they make you feel good. When you feel good, you allow the body to work properly in all areas. You allow it to perform as it naturally would.

IV.

If you were to live in a natural world free from the pressures and in-fluences of your society, you would have no need for clothes (other than protection from the elements). In a natural world, if the weather was nice, you would run around naked all day. You would not judge your body or anyone else's body. You would not feel embarrassment or shame. You would accept the look of your body no matter what it looked like. You would not compare yourself with others because you would know that you are unique and that you chose your specific body. If you chose your body so that it would carry you on your trajectory toward whatever you wanted to explore, then you would trust that you made the right choice.

Imagine being an astronaut and wearing a space suit. You are flying on a mission to Mars. With you on the trip are several other astronauts, all with specific jobs to perform. The captain wears a different suit than the biologist. Their suits are each specifically designed for their unique set of duties and responsibilities. The captain doesn't judge the biologist's suit to be better or worse because she knows that each suit matches each person's role on the ship.

Your body is your space suit. It was specifically designed for you based on the life you intended to live prior to your birth. Your natural height, sex, weight, skin color, and shape were all intended to give you the best possibility to explore the life you wanted to explore. It was an intention made with great care and thought.

If you believe your body is wrong for you, you are denying the intention you made prior to your birth. You must remember that your perspective is limited. Prior to your birth, you saw how your life might unfold from a much higher, wiser, and broader perspective. Your body is not wrong now and has never been wrong. You might allow it to evolve into something you prefer, but it is not wrong as it is now. The only way it could ever get better is by feeling better.

A good-feeling body is different than a good-looking body. How you feel in your body has to do with its energy and vitality, not with how it looks. If you think you would feel better if your body looked better, well, maybe that's true. But that has to do with your issues around worthiness, not about the shape of your body. All your body needs to function properly is your love. When you love (accept) your body as it is, you allow all the cells to allow well-being to flow. When you hate (fear) your body, you cause inner conflict and stress on the cells.

If you can believe that you chose your body for the role it would play in your life and for its contribution toward your trajectory, then you can appreciate your body as it is right now. If you can believe that your mind has the power to shape your body, then from your position of love, acceptance, and appreciation, your body can begin to take a shape you prefer. If you can believe that it's not how your body looks that's important, but rather how it feels, then you can move in the direction of a better-feeling body.

Your beliefs contribute to the creation of your reality. By increasing the intensity of beneficial beliefs, you bring what you want into your reality. By consciously choosing to analyze your limiting beliefs and reducing their intensity, you reduce fear and bring in more love. The modification of your belief system will change your experience of life. As you move away from limiting, fear-based beliefs toward loving, beneficial beliefs, your life and your body will begin to resemble what you prefer. It is simply a matter of practicing conscious creation utilizing the forces of the universe.

Chapter Four

Mind Power Versus Will Power

Your body sends you signals and feedback in the form of cravings, pains, hunger pangs, and many other feelings all day, every day. You are designed to respond to the messages your body is sending you. Your body will let you know when to wake, when to eat, when to relieve yourself, when to rest, and when to eat. It sends you the signals and you then take the action the body is requesting. Your body will not act without you. You control your body.

If your body is hungry, it sends you a signal in the form of hunger, which is an unpleasant feeling. In order to relieve this feeling, you must eat. What you eat is not so important. The pang will be relieved as long as you eat something. Now, keep in mind that you can also eat for pleasure, even if the body has not yet sent a signal to eat. When you have eaten too much, your body sends you a message in the form of an unpleasant feeling. If you eat any more, the feeling gets worse. As long as you don't eat any more, the feeling of being stuffed will go away as your body processes the food. This is how the system is designed.

When you feel an unpleasant feeling, you are supposed to notice it and take action to correct it. If you touch a hot stove, you feel pain, and you must take some action to relieve the pain so you remove your hand from the stove. The message the body is sending instructs you to take some action so that the pain (or unpleasant feeling) is removed. This system insures your health and survival.

You are designed to relieve the unpleasant feeling associated with any physical bodily condition. If you need to relieve yourself, you will feel an unpleasant feeling until you do so. If you need sleep, you will feel more and more tired until you sleep. Once you've taken the required action, you feel relief. The feeling of relief (a pleasant feeling) replaces the unpleasant feeling. You are supposed to feel good and when something comes up and you feel an unpleasant feeling, you are supposed to take action and return to your normal state of feeling good.

This is true of all unpleasant feelings, both physical and emotional. If you feel sad, you are supposed to choose a new perspective, soothe yourself, reach for better feeling thoughts, or do something to make yourself feel better. Hopefully, you will choose a mental action available within yourself that will ease your sadness and return you to your normal state of well-being. However, you might find temporary relief outside yourself. You might feel sad and reach for a drink, a drug, a smoke, or a piece of cake. These exterior sources of relief are limited in their effectiveness and seldom help in the long term. Typically, you feel worse for having succumbed to things you know don't benefit you.

In a normal, healthy body free from outside influences and pressures, you receive rather obvious signals from your body. You eat when hungry, you don't overeat, you sleep when tired, you wake when rested, you have energy, you feel good, you're alert and responsive, and, best of all, your waste elimination system performs like clockwork. Free of stress, the signals get through and you take the appropriate action at the right time.

However, in this world, you don't always receive the signals or take the appropriate action at the right time. You often eat when not hungry or choose to ignore your hunger pangs. By the time you do eat, you're either very hungry and you overeat, or you're tired and you simply eat what's available. When you're on a diet, you often try to endure the hunger pangs and skip eating altogether. This is typically ineffective and unnecessary. By messing around with how your system works, you interfere with the normal operations of many other systems. Your eating habits affect your sleep, your thinking, your elimination system, and many other vital systems.

By ignoring your body's signals, you alter how your body functions and the reception quality of those signals in the future. It throws the whole system off balance. Signals get lost or their message is unclear. You might receive an emotional feeling and mistake it for a hunger pang. You might become convinced that emotional pains are relieved the same way hunger pangs are relieved: by eating.

When you feel some emotional pain, such as sadness, frustration, anger, jealousy, despair, sorrow, anxiety, fear, or any other negative emotion, and you soothe yourself by eating, you don't solve the issue. You are meant to find a way to soothe your emotional pain mentally. You are meant to look inside yourself for relief. The emotion is a message telling you that you're looking at the subject from a perspective that does not serve you. You are meant to analyze the feeling and find relief by lowering the intensity of a fear. You are not meant to soothe yourself by looking outside yourself.

However, it is easier today to reach for something that's readily available. In the past, food was not so available and people could not easily pop something in their mouths to feel better. Now snacks are all around you everywhere you go. In the past, people might drink or smoke or fight or use some other means to feel better. Today, food is the easiest thing you can use. When you understand what is happening when you feel the urge to soothe yourself through food, you can stop and take a second thought before you take that first bite.

II.

In order to stop eating to soothe your negative emotions, you must find a set of mental tools that will do the trick. There are several tools you can use that will help you find relief. Not only is it better for your body to use a mental tool rather than to reach for food, but it is better for your emotional health and well-being as well. You are meant to take a new look at the issue that causes emotional pain from another perspective and when you find the right perspective, you will feel relief.

Here's how this works:

When you decide you want something, you set the universe in motion. The instant you birth a desire, the universe starts creating it and bringing it to you. You can ask for anything; it doesn't matter to the universe. Anything you ask for is on its way to you. There's nothing you need to do other than change your vibration. Your vibration allows you to perceive everything in your reality. If it's in your reality now, if you can perceive it now, it's because your vibration matches it. If it does not exist in your reality, it's because you are not yet a match to it. Once you get within the vibrational range of that thing you want, it enters your reality. This is simply the design of the system.

There's really nothing for you to do to change your own vibration. Your vibration is made up of a set of feelings, thoughts, beliefs, and expectations. When these things change, your reality changes. Now, you can't really, truly change your beliefs on your own. Experience helps to change beliefs. Once you've experienced something, the impact of that experience often causes a change in the structure of your beliefs if you're open to it. Some people are not open to changing their beliefs and so their lives don't really change either. In order to receive something new that you want, you must be open to modifying your belief system.

Whether you're open to changing your beliefs or not, if you've birthed a desire, the universe will place you in situations that are designed to alter your beliefs. These situations are called manifestation events. A manifestation event occurs every time you feel emotion. There are positive manifestation events and negative ones. When you feel a positive emotion, that manifestation event is working to raise the intensity and fully support a highly beneficial belief.

When you encounter any negative emotion, this is a manifestation event that is attempting to change some limiting belief. Since negative emotion is an unpleasant feeling, these events often feel unpleasant. You will think that something bad has happened. However, nothing bad has happened; it's just that from your perspective, you are encountering something that scares you and negative emotion arises to alert you to this irrational fear. There is some limiting belief based in an irrational fear that causes you to feel negative emotion.

You feel bad and your first thought is to soothe the bad feeling. At this point, you can ignore the event and reach for something to soothe yourself, or you can look at the event and analyze it. What caused the negative emotion? Why did you feel bad? What is the limiting belief? What is the fear behind the limiting belief? Is the fear irrational, meaning the source of the fear is not life-threatening? Is the fear a real fear, or is it false? Can you prove it's false? Can you look at the situation from another perspective and find relief? Once you've analyzed the fear and proven it's false, do you feel better?

This is the art of analysis. When you feel negative emotion, it is your signal that something is going on that brings up some fear. By analyzing it rather than ignoring it, you cause a change to your belief system. Instead of reaching for a cookie, you think about it and find evidence to prove the fear is false. If the fear is irrational, it is false. When you can prove to yourself it's false by finding evidence, you will lower the intensity of the limiting belief. This causes a shift in your belief system and your reality changes as a result. This is how you get everything you want.

When you ignore a negative emotion and resist the situation by calling it wrong or bad, you cause inner conflict and stress on the body. When you refuse to see it from another perspective or find evidence to prove it's false, you cause more stress because you're resisting the message. The stress feeds on itself and grows. You form a habit. It could be smoking, drinking, eating, or a combination of things. Habits are strengthened by momentum. The more often you do it, the more rigid and compelling the habit becomes. However, every single cell in your body seeks well-being and balance. You can get back to a balanced body relatively quickly.

If you've been reaching for a snack to soothe your negative emotions for your entire life, you can return to a balanced body within weeks. The momentum of a life-long habit can be reversed in just a few short weeks. This is due to the amazing restorative qualities of the body. Once you engage change, your cells respond by realigning themselves and balance is achieved. All it takes is a commitment to focus.

III.

Focus is the mental practice of keeping your thoughts in alignment with your desires. When you focus on something you really want, you can move around or side step everyday distractions. An urge may pop up, but you quickly ignore it and think about your desire. Typically, very strong desires encourage strong focus. If you want something badly enough, you're not easily taken off track by physical urges.

Focus is quite different than will power. Will power is the act of fighting against bodily urges by suppressing them and arguing against them. This fight causes you to focus on the urge, not the desire. When you fight against something, you bring your attention to it, and due to the Law of Attraction, it grows more and more and bigger and stronger until you can no longer fight it and you simply give in.

Focus places all your attention on the desire. The desire is so big that it is easy to think about it because the thought of it is so enjoyable. You'll do anything to achieve the desire. When an urge comes along, or some other distraction, you pay no attention to it and turn your attention back toward the desire. The urge will seem silly. Of course, you will not succumb to the urge. That would make no sense at all.

Can you see the difference here? Focus on your desire or focus on your urge. It's up to you. If you can maintain your focus on the desire, the desire will manifest. If you are distracted by the urge, the urge will win and your desire will be kept out of reach.

Imagine your desire is to win a body-building contest. This is your ultimate dream and nothing is more important to you. You work out in the gym twice daily. You are completely focused on everything you eat. In fact, with every bite of purely healthy food, you feel like you're moving toward your goal. You have friends and family who act as coaches and cheerleaders eagerly supporting you every step of the way. Whenever you do anything, you think about achieving your dream. You fully intend to win the competition and you fully expect to hold the trophy and hear the cheers.

When you work out, you feel the body's urge to rest and you do not give it a second thought. Instead, you think about how your body will feel when you win the competition. Your body sends you the urge to eat an ice cream sundae and you snicker. Instead, you reach for a satisfying protein shake. Your body sends you a thought to take it easy and watch some TV. Instead, you go out for a jog. Every time your body sends you a strong signal in the form of an urge, you turn it around and find something that helps you move toward your goal. Your focus allows you to turn your attention away from the urge and back to your desire. The strong desire makes focusing easy and enjoyable and in doing so removes the power of the urge. It all comes from a positive emotional state of being.

Now imagine you have worked very hard to get in shape for this competition. You have sacrificed a lot including a lot of your favorite foods and fun with friends. But you've gotten yourself in great shape and now you're ready to compete. You begin the competition and realize there are a lot of people here who are in very good shape and you begin to doubt your chances. Ultimately, you do not win the competition. You feel great disappointment and frustration. Maybe this dream is not possible for you.

Maybe you should give up. Now, when the urge comes to eat or watch TV or something else, you find it more powerful. It's not as easy to turn your focus back to your goal. The urge is calling to you and because of your diminished emotional state of being, you succumb.

Your lowered emotional state of being allows for the stronger influence of the urge and you give in. All the momentum created by months of focus and work has now stopped and a new momentum is starting. If you give up on your dream, you'll likely give in to those urges. However, as soon as you decide to pursue your dream despite the results of this last competition, you regain your focus and start building momentum once again.

IV.

The power of the mind is an awesome thing to behold. Focus brings the full energy of the mind onto the subject of your attention. When aligned with what you really want and who you really are, the mind engages and leverages universal forces. When you are focused on something you want, the entire universe is there working with you. It might be difficult for you to comprehend, but that is how the system was designed. When you focus strongly on what is wanted, the universe stands with you and the power that created the universe is channeled through you.

It might not seem like you have this ability. From where you stand now, you may have never really focused that strongly on any single desire. Sure, you might have achieved some small goals in the past, but that big dream still eludes you. Why can't you manifest that big dream? Why are you unable to leverage the forces of the universe to achieve that goal? It all has to do with one thing: fear.

Fear derails your efforts. Fear arises in the form of doubt and disbelief. When you don't believe something is possible, it becomes impossible for you. However, nothing is inherently impossible. If you can conceive it, it can be achieved. If you have doubt, you disengage the powers of the universe and without them, you stand alone. When you are focused on your dream and aligned with that desire, you have no doubt. You know it will come. When you engage this level of focus, you leverage universal energies and this alignment creates miracles. When you really want something, you must remove doubt. Doubt is fear; faith is love. You want to move from fear to love, from doubt to faith (or knowing or belief), and the alignment engages universal power. Your wildest dreams can be achieved if you will only trust that your full faith, focus, and belief brings with it a power you cannot begin to imagine.

When you believe that it is all up to you alone to create anything you desire, whether that is a lean body, a loving relationship, a new house, a dream job or business, you set up a perspective that allows for the possibility of failure. If it's all up to you then you create the possibility for failure. Failure only becomes a possibility when you have doubt. Without doubt, you could not fail. Here again, your beliefs play an important role in creating your reality.

If you believed you could not fail, you would engage the forces of the universe and together you would be so powerful, so aligned, so confident, so effective, that you could not fail. It would simply be out of the realm of possibility. The universe yields to you. When you act in faith, trusting that things will ultimately go your way, without any doubt or fear, with clarity of focus, you can achieve anything. Losing a few pounds is nothing compared to the power you possess.

When you look back on any perceived failure in the past, you can observe two important points. One, you thought you were doing it all on your own. You did not understand that you were fully supported by your inner self, your inner guides, and the full force and power of the universe. And two, you can see that at some point, doubt crept in. You might have been on your way to achieving your dream, but as soon as some fear presented itself, doubt caused the dream to unravel.

If you can get yourself to believe that you create your own reality, that you have a vast inner support network to back you, that the universe yields to your desires, and that the power of focus aligns all your support behind you with one mission in mind, you can absolutely be, have, and do anything you desire in this reality. It is the basic design of the system. Everyone has the power. Anyone can achieve their dreams. There is just one thing you have to remember in order to fully engage all of this information:

You are worthy of anything you desire.

Chapter Five

You Are Worthy of Anything You Desire

If you have read anything we have previously written, you have heard us say that you are as worthy as any who have ever or will ever live. You are exactly as worthy as anyone else on the planet. Your value is identical to everyone you know and everyone who exists right now. The fact that you are worthy means that you can have, be, and do anything you desire in this playground called physical reality.

You are a unique expression of source. You are here to explore reality from a unique perspective. No other person has ever or will ever perceive reality as you are perceiving it right now. You are completely and absolutely unique to all the universe. Your unique experience of life adds to the sum total of the universe since each point of perspective is equally unique and all points of perspective are equally valid and valuable, one not more so than any other. Your complete and total uniqueness proves your worthiness and value to all that is.

If you can birth a desire, you can achieve that desire. There's nothing more to it than that. Once you've birthed the desire, you either allow it to come to you or resist it. Once you birth a desire, the universe finds a way to bring it to you. If you allow it to come, by going with the flow and not fighting against things, it will come. If you are constantly arguing with the conditions, you are resisting what you want.

You are worthy of all that you want. Your doubt that you are worthy is what causes much of your resistance. Fear and self-doubt are resistant in nature. Love, confidence, and ease are allowing in nature. When you experience self-doubt, you are feeling unworthy. When you experience confidence, you are feeling worthy. Worthy-feeling people allow what they want to flow to them. Unworthy-feeling people resist it because they fear receiving that which they are not worthy of.

You may feel worthy. You might consider yourself to be confident. But if you are resisting anything, there is a little unworthiness in there. Remove some of those feelings of unworthiness and you will begin to allow more to come to you. How do you come to actually know your own worthiness? You adopt a higher perspective on your life.

You are an eternal and limitless being of pure positive love. You are love. That's who you are. That's who everyone is. You are all part of source and source is pure love. Who you really are is a being of love. Who you are being right now, in your home, in your body, is something less than that. You are moving from who you are right now, to who you really are. You are an eternal and limitless being of pure positive love.

When you transition to the nonphysical, you will reemerge as a being of pure positive love. You will return to the fullest and broadest expression of who you really are. You will shed all your fear and regain pure love and acceptance.

In physical reality, your path is one of moving from a fear-based being to a love-based being. You are in the process of moving from fear to love. You have done this many, many times in countless other lives. In this life, you are closer to being who you really are than in any other life. It is a progression from one life to the next. You are becoming more conscious and self-aware. Everyone is on the journey to becoming who they really are. Some are fighting it and others are progressing with ease and joy.

Who you think you are is not who you are. This is due to the structure of physical reality. You have an identity. We call it your persona. Your ego guards against the loss or injury of the persona just as the survival instinct guards against the loss or injury of the body. The ego tries to protect the persona. It is a survival mechanism.

In the past, long, long ago, one's persona was really very basic and the ego was not so pronounced. Times were simpler then and when one lived in a very small and tight-knit community, one's persona was not very fragile, because all knew where they stood in their community. Today, your society is quite large and advanced. You now have opportunities where few existed in historic times. You are not bound by the restraints of a closed society but are free to explore your world as you please. Never before in the history of your society have so many been offered so many options and opportunities. In this society, your persona becomes quite fragile and your ego must work hard to protect it.

You see yourself as a success or failure, as intelligent or not, as a good parent, lover, child, friend, employee, boss, etc. You identify with your career, your education, your race and color, your possessions, your mate, etc. Yet none of these things have anything to do with who you really are. They are all part of the persona you have developed and nothing more. They do not represent the real you. They are all aspects of the real you but are diminished due to irrational fear. Your ego uses irrational fear to protect the persona.

If you consider yourself to be polite and proper, you would react negatively if someone were to infer that you were being rude. The ego wants to protect your view of yourself. Since you view yourself as polite, being considered rude is an affront against your persona. Your ego instills fear and you react to that fear by adopting a limiting perspective and as a result, you feel negative emotion. Since you see yourself in a certain light, you cannot be wrong, for that would jeopardize your persona. So you attack the person who called you rude and make them wrong. This is how many fights are started.

If you recognized that you are a being of pure positive love, not the false edifice of your persona, your ego could not be bruised. If you knew you were a being of love, then nothing could be done to embarrass, anger, or sorrow you. Your ego would fade into the background because it would serve no purpose. When you live as a being of love, you are without fear. Since ego uses fear, your ego would have nothing to use.

You are not your persona. You are not really who you think you are. You are far more than that. You have far more to offer. You are far more powerful than you think. You are as worthy as any who have ever lived and you have the ability to access infinite intelligence and leverage the powers of the universe in any way you see fit. You are the creator of your life and you can adopt complete control over the quality of your life. You are responsible for everything in your reality. There is no fate or luck; it is all created by you. You have all the power.

You are not your persona and you are not your body. Your body is the vehicle you use to navigate physical reality. It is your physical space suit. Without it you could not be physical. You are a nonphysical being experiencing physicality through your body. You can see your body when you look in the mirror, but if you are not your body, where are you? You are within all the cells of your body. You are the source of energy that enlivens the cells of your body. You are the conductor of the orchestra that is your body. You are the captain of the ship that is your body. You are the leader of the community of trillions of cells that make up your body. But you are not your body.

Your body is a representation of your thoughts, feelings, beliefs, and expectations, but it is not you. You can control certain functions of the body consciously, but the vast majority of its functions are done without your awareness. Your body is comprised of individual cells and each cell is an individual point of consciousness, just as alive as you are. Each cell seeks well-being just as you do. Each cell is here to live a joyful and expansive existence, just as you are.

So then, you are worthy, you are unique, you are not your persona but something greater, you are not your body, but you are the creator of your body, there is no fate, and you are the creator of your reality. There is no coincidence, no luck, no randomness; everything happens for a reason and a purpose. You have a vibration and that vibration brings forth that which you focus your attention on. This is an attractive universe; nothing can be pushed away. Now that you understand all that, how does it apply to your desire to create a lean and healthy body?

II.

You believe that you are your body and that your body is a representation of you. It is to an extent. You believe that if you can make your body look better, it will reflect better on you, you'll feel better, and then you'll actually be better. In other words. if you had a better body, you would feel more worthy. Your idea of your own worthiness has a lot to do with the condition and attractiveness of your body (or job, or mate, or money in the bank). However, we have explained that you are already worthy and so when you seek to do something in order to achieve a feeling of worthiness, it doesn't ever work. Your life is a reflection of your current feelings of self-worth. Your body is a reflection of your current feelings of self-worth. Your entire life, including your home, friends, bank account, career, etc., is a reflection of your feelings of worthiness. Increase your feelings of worthiness first and everything else will improve.

Nothing you do will really affect your feeling of worthiness when you are doing it just for the goal of feeling better about yourself. You may lose ten pounds and feel better for a while, but then the self-doubt and insecurity manifests in some situation and you go back to feeling how you felt before and the weight comes back as well. It is the feeling of worthiness that controls everything in your life, including your weight. It is not the food you eat. If you felt worthy, you would be inspired to eat, sleep, drink, and exercise in a way that matched how you felt about yourself. The inspiration comes from your feelings about yourself. The inspiration causes you to act. The quality of inspiration you receive depends on how you feel about yourself. It's all about the feeling.

If you did not feel worthy, you would not act like a person who knew their own worthiness. Your thoughts would be different. The words you spoke would be different. Your actions would be different. Your attitude, level of confidence, and approach to life would be different. You would actually see yourself differently. Because you see yourself differently than someone who knows their own worth, you make different choices.

Let's imagine for a moment that you felt perfectly and absolutely worthy. Imagine if you knew you were as worthy (yet no more worthy) as anyone else on the planet. Imagine you understood that the version of you that exists now is perfect in every way. You might change in the future to another version of you, but the one who exists in this moment could not be any more perfect. If you knew this, you would approach your life in a totally different manner.

If you knew your worth, you would not make choices that did not fully align with who you know yourself to be. If you knew you were the creator of your own reality, you would not say things that did not align with who you are. If you understood your power, you would not settle for something less than the highest and most elegant manifestation of what you wanted. If you understood your perfection (and the whole idea of perfection), you would not discount any aspect of yourself and you would never compare yourself to anyone else.

Let's talk about the concept of perfection. We say that if you would not change any aspect of something, you would call that thing perfect. If you looked at a work of art by Picasso and would not change anything about it, you would call it perfect the way it is. Does the painting resemble anything you previously would have considered perfect? Why are the ears out of place and why is there a nose coming out of the head in that spot? It doesn't seem to make sense. In fact, if the works of Picasso were created just thirty years earlier, they would not have been valued at all. The people of more modern times were able to see the perfection in Picasso's work. Their vibrations had risen to that level.

In the future, people will understand the concept of perfection and will realize that every person is perfect as they are in the moment. Life constantly evolves and changes. You change billions of times per second. You are constantly changing. Each and every cell in your body is changing. You cannot help but to change. It is part of life. However, in this very moment, you are perfect just as you are.

You are the perfect representation of your vibration just as you are. You stand at the perfect place to embark on a new path toward a new desire, just as you are. Your entire life has led up to this moment in time. If you are reading this now, you have reached a vibrational level high enough to resonate with this material. If you want to change the shape of your body, you have lived a life that has unfolded perfectly to create this desire and you have the ability to see it through to its ultimate manifestation.

III.

You do not want a lean body. What you want is to feel good. You do not want money, love, a career, or things. What you really want is to feel good. This is a feeling reality. All you are ever doing is either feeling good or not so good. Nothing is more important than how you feel. If you felt good right now, wouldn't that be nice? If you felt wonderful right now, what would be better than that? When you want something, it's not the thing you want, it's the feeling you think that thing will bring.

The funny thing about feeling good is that you often choose not to feel good until the thing you want actually manifests. Unfortunately, that's not how the system was designed. You are meant to feel good and from the high vibrational frequency of feeling good, other good feelings come your way. Your feelings attract conditions that match them. When you wish for something in order to feel good and you choose to feel bad until it comes, you are actually attracting the conditions that match how you feel. You simply cannot get to what you want by feeling bad. You can't get a lean body by feeling bad about the body you have now. It will not work.

In order to allow what you want to flow to you, you must appreciate the positive aspects of that specific subject and use these things to make your-self feel good about the subject. For instance, let's say you want a better job. If you choose to hate your job and you quit, you might find another job, but that job will feel the same as the old job. The new job will match your feelings. What you hated in the old job will eventually show up in the new job too. Your feelings inform your vibration and your vibrational signal goes out into the universe and brings back a match.

If you focus on what you consider to be a negative aspect of your body, such as fat, your feelings influence your vibration to such a degree that the universe will reinforce those feelings. You will actually be given plenty of examples that you are indeed fat. You will hear comments, you will inter-pret looks, you will feel exposed, you will imagine that people are looking at you, talking about you, and thinking bad thoughts about you. Your per-ception of reality will match how you feel. It will reinforce your negative feelings and this will lower your emotional state of being. From this low emotional state of being, you will be given inspiration to make you feel better, but that inspiration will not be in alignment with the worthy being you are. It will not be in alignment with the perfect person you are. It will be aligned with your perception of yourself in the moment.

If you feel worthy, you have access to thoughts, ideas, and inspiration that match how you feel about yourself. If you feel worthy, you will likely maintain a high emotional state of being. If you understand your per-fection, you will not slip so easily into a lower emotional state of being. When you realize your worthiness and your perfection as you are right now in this very moment, you will feel good more and more of the time. Feeling good aligns with the forces of the universe. Feeling good brings you into the state of allowing. Feeling good creates an environment where the universe matches how you feel with what you get. Feeling good opens the door to everything you want.

So then, how does feeling good make it easier to lose weight and keep the weight off? How does feeling good increase your chances of losing weight and creating a healthy and lean body in the process? How can you even feel good when you don't like the shape of your body as it is right now? Let us explain this in more detail.

This is an attractive universe, not a resistant one. You attract what you want (or don't want) by your focus of attention. If you don't like your body as it is now, you tend to think about, complain about, and be ashamed about the things you don't like. As you place your focus on these things, the universe via the Law of Attraction brings more of what you don't like. When you feel bad, you receive thoughts that resonate with this low emotional state. You have control over the thoughts you think, but you don't practice that control and so the thoughts that come to you are aligned with that which you do not want.

You think that if you can pick out something wrong with your body (or your life) and fix it or change it, everything will be better. So you endure hunger and you use some will power and you lose a few pounds. But the result of this doesn't allow you to feel good for very long because you haven't addressed the main issue. You are being resistant to what is and you are trying to destroy the aspect of your body that you hate. You are trying to push it away. You are fighting against it and losing the battle. You are resisting it, but it is still there. This approach is futile in an attractive universe.

The only way to get anything you want is to allow it to come. The only way to allow anything to come is by creating an environment where it's easy to allow. Are you allowing when you are hating the fat? No, you are resisting. Are you allowing when you are ashamed of your body? No. You are resisting. Are you allowing when you are starving yourself? No, you are resisting. We understand that you want to perform some action to solve your problem, but the effort involved will never yield the results you want. When you take action just to solve a problem, you do it alone. Uninspired action does not engage the leverage of universal forces. Action against something you think is bad only reinforces the bad. It only makes it stronger.

We are purposely repeating ourselves here because this concept is so counter-intuitive and so against the grain of your instincts that we must reinforce our message. You believe that action solves problems, but it doesn't. Uninspired action never yields the results you truly desire and it often makes the problem much worse. The key to receiving anything you want is to get yourself into a state of acceptance, understand that there is nothing wrong, appreciate the positive aspects of the situation, and focus on something wanted in a holistic way. Then, once you've gotten this approach all set up and you're focused on feeling good, you will be inspired to action that will utilize the forces of the universe and each step will be pleasurable.

Let's return to a real-life example. You have found yourself with a body that does not feel good. You are not as fit as you would like to be. You are not as lean as you would prefer. You look at others and compare yourself unfavorably. You don't want to wear a swimsuit. You can't fit into your clothes and you don't want to buy larger clothes. And you certainly don't want to be seen naked. So from this position in life you birth a desire to lose weight.

The problem seems simple: lose twenty pounds and everything will be right again. However, there's more to it than that. If you had been feeling good, you would not have gained the weight. If you had been free of stress, you would not have gained the weight. If you had been feeling worthy, you would not have added those twenty pounds. The fact is that you didn't accidentally eat a lot of cheesecake and put on a few pounds. Something in your life caused you to feel bad enough for long enough so that the weight was attracted. The weight is a sign of resistance.

You might argue that weight gain is a normal part of the aging process. We would agree that in your society it seems to be normal for people to gain weight as they get older. It is not. What's normal is the increased effects of stress and worry. What's normal is the slow regression of how you feel. You felt better when you were younger. You don't feel as good now. You are allowing the illusion of reality to get the best of you. You are paying more attention to things you don't like and less attention to things you do like.

We will ask you a few questions. Are there more grumpy old people or grumpy young people? Do adults giggle? Are adults silly? Who is more giddy with joy, the old or the young? In a natural world, free from the pressures of your modern society, you would know your worthiness and you would feel joy every day. These two attributes would keep you lean.

Now we will ask again: is it more effective to use will power to lose the weight and keep it off, or is it better to know your worthiness and to feel good?

IV.

We think it is a good time for us to explain our perspective to you. We, Joshua, are a group of nonphysical teachers. We exist in the nonphysical realm, yet we are very much focused on your lives here in the physical realm. We enjoy sharing our perspective with you. We enjoy teaching. We are thrilled to be a part of this fascinating conversation. But who are we really?

Imagine a room with several people collectively writing a book together. Everyone puts forth an idea and together we reach a consensus on every word. All of us have experienced many lives in physical reality and we want to use our knowledge of universal forces and the mechanism of physical reality to assist you in experiencing life to the fullest. Now, instead of picturing several of us in a room all working together to form this book of information, imagine several hundred people in a theater. Now imagine several thousand people in an arena. Now imagine a football stadium filled with people all working together to share their ideas and collaborate on this book. Now imagine all of the football stadiums in the world filled with people all working together. This would be a small fraction of the amount of intelligent energy being put forth to write this one book.

We see your world, your lives, your trials and tribulations from a much higher, broader perspective. It is a perspective that you cannot know. It is quite different from your perspective. There are discoveries that will be made that will allow people to gain a higher perspective. However, from where you sit right now, all you can do is imagine what the higher perspective looks like. This is a perfectly valid notion. If you can remove yourself from your limited perspective and imagine what a higher perspective might look like, you'll make huge strides toward achieving your dreams.

If you look back on historic times, you can easily see that the perspectives of people who lived then were much more limited than your own. They once believed the world was flat. They did not understand the law of gravity. They did not believe that the earth revolved around the sun. They could not imagine that man would one day travel to any spot on the planet within a few short hours. They could not conceive of the computer or the internet. Their perspective was limited.

In ancient times, people believed that if they sailed too far, they would fall off the side of the earth. You believe that in order to lose weight, you must control your eating through will power. Both of these beliefs are limited. From our perspective, we understand that there is great joy to be found in food. It is one of the aspects of physical reality that we miss the most. You cannot gain through pain or suffering. You gain through joy. Everything you want comes through feeling good. When you feel bad, you can be sure that you are moving away from that which you desire.

Certainly you can take action to create minor, temporary results. However, action inspired from a negative emotional state of being yields paltry results that tend to fade over time. You cannot get around the fact that it's your approach to life that creates your reality, not your actions. Your approach to life, whatever that may be, is the tracks on which the great locomotive travels. You can slow down or speed up the train, but you can't change its course. The train will always go wherever the tracks take it. There is no steering wheel on a train. In order to change its course, you must lay new tracks. We are going to show you how to lay new tracks. We are going to talk about a new approach to life in general. It is from this new approach that you will achieve easy and long-lasting results.

It does not matter what has happened in the past. Your perspective on past events clouds the reality of those events anyway. Your memory is foggy at best. What happened then has no effect on your current reality in this moment unless you allow it to. You don't need to rehash or solve any problem of the past. You are alive now and from this point in time, anything is possible. The only things standing in your way are limiting beliefs tied to past events. Reduce the intensity of limiting beliefs as they arise in the moment and you will move up the vibrational scale to a state of ease and allowing.

Everything in your life has brought you to this moment in time. You are in the perfect place at the perfect time with the perfect state of mind. You are open to new ideas. You are receiving guidance from infinite intelligence. You are expanding and increasing the intensity of beneficial beliefs. You are on the verge of a wonderful and exciting new life. Nothing can hold you back except you. You hold the key. Will you stay where you are or will you use your key to unlock the door that's right in front of you? If you choose to stay where you are, we fully understand. It's safe there. Your ego is telling you not to change. Your ego is trying to make you doubt our words. But you understand these words. They make sense to you. You know that what we are saying has truth within it. You are ready for the next step. Take your key and unlock that door and together we will go where your dreams live.

Chapter Six

Your Approach To Life and How To Change It

Momentum is a topic we love to talk about. There is positive momentum that keeps what you want coming to you and there is negative momentum that creates this need to talk about and complain about all the things you don't like. We get it. It's how you were raised. It's the example set by your parents, your teachers, your news media, and even your leaders. Your friends love to gossip. Everyone likes to look at the train wreck. You are titillated by controversy and personal tragedy. Yet, you are not understanding what you are doing. By thinking about things you do not like, you bring more of that into your life. By talking about the things you think are bad or wrong, you are encouraging the momentum of that vibration to remain in your life. Nothing is bad. Nothing is wrong. It just is.

This is an attractive universe. Everything comes to you. Everything is neutral. You choose what comes by paying attention to it. You decide what is good or bad by your choice of perspective. If you choose a limited perspective, you will see how wrong something is. However, when you choose to look at something from the higher perspective, you are choosing to see that it is not wrong after all. This is the approach to life that will create an atmosphere of allowing. When you are in the state of allowing (not doing), everything you want will begin to flow to you.

There is no wrong anywhere in the universe. Anything you perceive to be wrong is simply an illusion created by your limited perspective. Choose the higher perspective and you will see it is right. Everything is right. If you can understand that there is no wrong, that everything is right, and that you have a choice over which perspective you think is more empowering for you, then you will have chosen an approach to life that serves you.

All we are suggesting is that reality is in the eye of the beholder. That is the truth. How you see your reality is actually how it is. You allow yourself to get caught up in the stress and drama of everyday life. However, it is your fear that creates the stress. It's your irrational fear, not anyone else's. You choose to worry. You choose to look far into the future. You choose to imagine the worst possible outcome. You choose to feel unfortunate, unlucky, unblessed, unloved, etc. You choose to compare yourself to others unfavorably. You choose to view your life from a perspective that doesn't serve you. What you must understand is that none of that is real. You're making it all up. It may seem real and you may be completely fooled by the illusion, but it's simply not reality. Your reality is whatever you choose it to be.

We hear you saying, "Wait a minute, Joshua. I see my body. I see the conditions around me. I see my bank account. I see all these things. They are real. How can you say it's only my perception?"

Excellent question. Let us explain.

Imagine yourself as a child. You came into this life full of joy and love. That's all you packed for your trip to Earth. You did not pack fear, doubt, worry, regret, resentment, frustration, or remorse. You packed joy and love. When you were a child, you thought only of the day ahead. You did not project yourself too far into the future. You had fun in the day. You loved and felt as if you were loved in return. It was only when you got a little older that things started to change for you.

At some point in your childhood you started to feel less secure. You started to compare yourself to others. You started to worry. You started to wish things were different. At one point, early in your childhood, you chose a perspective that did not serve you. This caused negative emotion and you felt sad. Maybe you even cried. When you got over it, you felt relief.

However, you didn't really do anything to get over it. Time healed your wound. You took your mind off it and the perspective changed. A day passed and this was enough time to get to a higher perspective. At this point, you could have realized that your perspective either caused emotional pain or relieved it, depending on which perspective you chose. If you chose the limited perspective, you felt pain. If you chose the higher perspective, you felt relief. If you understood this simple fact of physical reality, you could have softened endless disappointments and heartbreak. Instead you chose another approach to life.

The approach to life you chose involved creating conditions that make you feel good. This is a much more difficult approach to life. Only dictators and despots have the ability to control their conditions long enough to make it work for them. And even then, it never works in the long term. You try to manipulate your parents, and siblings, and friends, and teachers into behaving in a way that allows you to feel good. And they are all doing the same to you. If they behave well, you feel good. If they do something you do not like, you feel bad. In order for you to feel good, you must control every aspect of their behavior. If you don't feel good, then they did something to upset you and that is wrong. If you feel good, then they did nothing to upset you and that is good.

How does one coerce the conditions so that they feel good? Let's look at your parents. They were nice to you when you behaved and so, for the most part, you behaved well. You conformed to their wishes, not yours. You got good grades at school. You did your chores. You chose mates that they would approve of. You changed who you were because you could not endure the emotional pain associated with their disapproval, judgment, or punishment. You conformed to their wishes for the sole purpose of avoiding negative emotion. That was a great sacrifice and it was completely unnecessary.

The same is true of your teachers. You conformed to their wishes in order to avoid the negative emotions associated with their disapproval. This caused you to worry for the first time. You worried about being late for school. You worried about being absent. You worried about getting bad grades. You worried about forgetting assignments, or losing papers, or a million other things. You worried that they would get angry with you and then tell your parents or embarrass you in front of your classmates. You lived up to their rules and expectations for the sole reason of avoiding any negative emotion because you never learned how to deal with it.

Your entire approach to life is dedicated to the sole purpose of avoiding negative emotion.

You want to lose weight not to feel good in a lean body, but to remove the negative emotion associated with the body you have now. From your limited perspective, you believe your body is wrong and you want to fix it. When you think of your body as wrong or bad, you feel negative emotion. What you are trying to do by losing the weight is not rid yourself of fat, it's simply to ease the pain of the negative emotion.

II.

Negative emotion is nothing to be afraid of. It is simply your built-in guidance system letting you know when you are focusing on something in a way that does not serve you. Think about the mechanism of physical reality. Why are you here in the first place? What is the purpose of experiencing physical reality? Because physical reality is tangible, it is different than the nonphysical. In physical reality you can experience feelings that are not available to you in the nonphysical realm.

In physical reality you can experience fear because it is part of the survival instinct. In the nonphysical realm there is no fear, because there is no need for fear. Fear is an integral part of physical reality, but it is completely absent in the nonphysical. So fear is a beneficial emotion in this plane of existence. It keeps you alive. When you focus on something that has the potential to do you harm, you receive an indication in the form of an emotion called fear. It is a warning that is felt on the inside. It is a message sent to you from the nonphysical.

Is an emotion physical or nonphysical? It's nonphysical. It has no mass or physical properties. It's like a thought or any other feeling. It exists in the physical world, but can only be felt by the person experiencing the emotion. When you feel fear, others may sense it, but no one knows really what you're experiencing. It is an individual thing. Some people feel fear intensely and others feel it less so. This is true of all emotions.

If you could not feel fear, you would do things that would likely lead to death or injury. You would leave this planet rather prematurely. You would not have the time to explore the things that interest you, because that exploration would probably lead to your death. That's why fear is such an important aspect of physical reality. Without fear, the mechanism would not function as it was intended.

Now that you understand that fear is a crucial element in the fabrication of physical reality, you must also realize that every other emotion has its purpose as well. All negative emotions are some form of fear. It does not matter how you label the emotion. If it doesn't feel good, it's fear. If it feels good, the emotion is some form of love. There are really only two emotions, fear and love. Fear lets you know when you're focused on something that has the potential to bring you something unwanted. The positive emotion of love lets you know that you're focused on something in a way that's aligned with what you want.

Now that you understand the role that emotions play in the creation of the life you desire, you can look at any emotion and realize it's a message. Let's look at the emotion you call regret. Regret is a negative emotion based in fear. What's the fear? It's the fear of loss. When you look back at some event that occurred in the past and you wish it had happened differently, you are experiencing the negative emotion of regret. Had things been done differently, you believe you would be better off. You fear that you lost something because of the outcome of the event. This is simply not true and that's why you feel the negative emotion.

In the case of regret, the fear is irrational. Why is it irrational? Because you did not die as a result of the event that you regret. Your life took a turn in a new direction because of the event, but you certainly did not die and so the fear is irrational. It is also irrational because had the event turned out differently than it did, your life would not have unfolded as it did. Since you cannot know what the other outcome might have led to, you are simply creating a story you're using to make yourself feel bad. You're creating the entire illusion. You might have died three days after the event. Something terrible may have happened if the event played out differently. But you choose a perspective that the actual result of the event was bad or wrong and in doing so you bring up this negative emotion called regret.

Can you see the message in the emotion? Can you see that the negative emotion is letting you know that this train of thought, this perspective you've chosen, is not serving you? Do you understand this? You have chosen to create a story that says something bad happened. However, nothing bad did happen. It all worked out. You're here, aren't you? You can't know where you might be right now if the event had led you on another path. You might be dead. You might be bankrupt. You might be alone. If you're going to make up a story, write one that makes you feel good, not bad.

If you choose a perspective that does not serve you, you will feel negative emotion every time. Isn't that an excellent system? It never fails. You might choose to ignore the emotion, but it will always be there, every single time. You cannot escape it, thank God. You can't turn it off. It is always on. Even in your dream state. It never fails you. Never ever. It's fail-safe.

Why would such a system be so reliable? Because it's so important. It's one of the most crucial aspects of physical reality. It is integral to the whole design. Without it, you could not create your own reality. You could not control the unfolding of your life. You could not achieve your dreams. Without your emotional guidance system, this reality would not work as intended. It would serve no purpose.

Your purpose in this life is to expand through experience and fulfill your desires in a joyous manner. You are here to explore. You are here to create desires. You are here to expand with every interest and every experience. You are here to bring forth new thoughts and new ideas. You are here to be a unique expression of source. You come to experience reality in a way that has never been experienced before. In doing so, you wanted guidance every step of the way.

When you think of some past experience, you have this feeling of regret. You wish it were different than it was. Would you agree that it is not helpful to wish that it were different? Since it has already happened, what is the purpose of that? How could wanting something that can't be changed be helpful in any way? It can't be. Once the moment has been created in your reality, you cannot change it. It cannot be changed. If it cannot be changed, then it is perfect. Why would you want to change something that's perfect? Because you still believe in the illusion that it could be changed. You still use your imagination to change it. You are looking at something that can't be changed and imagining that it might have been better. This use of your imagination does not serve you and your guidance system is telling you that by the feeling you call regret.

You are choosing to look at the past in a way that is actually at odds with what you want. If you continue to view your past in this manner, you will continue to experience the aspects of your life that you do not want. If you knew this going in, you would not look back at something and wish it were different. You would look forward to something from a perspective that aligns with what you do want. Doesn't that make complete sense? Isn't this a very excellent system? Aren't you glad physical reality is designed so well?

You feel the feeling of regret and as soon as you get the first inkling of this feeling, you realize that you're adopting a perspective on this past event that does not serve you. What do you do? You change your perspective. You reach for a higher perspective. As soon as you find one that brings forth the feeling of relief, you know you've returned your focus to what's wanted and away from what's unwanted. You stopped the momentum of the unwanted and you've reengaged the momentum toward what you do want. This is how you create your reality. You felt bad for an instant and you immediately searched for a different perspective until you felt relief. Therefore, the negative emotion barely registered and you felt bad for a very short period of time. In this case, the negative emotion was not such a bad thing.

But you don't choose your perspective on purpose, do you? You hold onto the limited perspective as long as you can. You let it roll around in your head and the negative emotion persists. It stays with you as long as you keep holding onto this perspective that does not serve you. Your emotional guidance never gives up. If you don't pay attention, it will only get stronger.

It's not the events that cause you to feel bad; it's your perspective. The things that bring up negative emotion for you are not bad things in and of themselves. They are just the way they are. They are neutral. It's you who decides if something is good or bad, right or wrong. You create your own reality by deciding to love something or someone or deciding to hate them. It is all up to you. You have the capacity to love anything and anyone, but you seem predisposed toward hating them. This is simply a knee-jerk response caused by fear.

Let's imagine that something happened in your childhood that you regret or resent. Let's say your parents got divorced and one of them moved out and you felt abandoned. You imagine that if they had stayed together, your life would be better. Now, you have no possible way of knowing that, yet you still insist on creating this story that does not serve you. If your parents stayed together, it is quite likely that your home life would be far more stressful than it actually was.

You make up these stories about how your life could have been better if only this or that would have happened. You resent anyone who contributed to an outcome that seemed like it was wrong. If your parents divorced each other when you were young, you may hold onto resentment for a very long time. You may hold one or both of them responsible for your unhappy childhood that created this problematic adulthood. However, you have no idea how it would have been had they remained married.

The thing to remember about your childhood is that you knew going in that the specific parents you chose would create an environment that would launch you on a trajectory toward what you came here to explore. You chose them knowing they would not stay married for very long. You chose them knowing they would move to the city where you were raised. You knew they would have or not have more children. You knew going in what your childhood would be like and you chose them because you knew that life in this family would cause you to birth some very specific desires.

You chose your family and the time and place of your birth along with your body because you knew that this environment would spur you onward to explore certain interesting aspects of physical reality. When you choose to look back in regret or resentment, you are saying to yourself that you made an error in judgment. The desires that were created out of the environment of your childhood set you seeking that which you came here to explore. If you blame others for helping you create these desires, you're missing the whole point. Everything has unfolded just as you knew it would. The only thing that is holding you back is your attachment to the wrongness of that environment. Help yourself by understanding that it was all planned and that it was all right.

III.

Your perspective is your story. You can tell a story that aligns with who you really are and what you really want or you can make up a story that conflicts with what you want. It's up to you. You can choose a perspective that's empowering or limited. It's your choice. You can choose to be engaged in the world around you or frozen with fear. It's your choice. Lean in and move through the fear and your self-imposed limitations will fade away.

If the fear is irrational, there's nothing real to fear. The fear is false. It might feel real, but like a movie, it's just an illusion. When it comes to irrational fear, the only thing you fear is the negative emotion that comes as a result of trying something new or something out of your comfort zone. As soon as you learn to deal with the fear, by shaping your own positive perception or by analyzing the fear itself, you no longer allow yourself to be limited.

Currently, you live a very limited life. Your experiences all fall within a zone of comfort. You fear the ramifications caused by negative emotion. You do not want to do anything, see anything, or talk to anyone where there is a potential for negative emotion. But what really causes the negative emotion in the first place? It's the way you choose to look at something. It's the way you choose to react to some event. You fear the emotion and you have no control over your perspective, so you have no control over the emotion itself. But what if you could release the negative emotion as soon as it started? What if negative emotion didn't really bother you? What if you could feel the negative emotion and still feel good? Then you would free yourself from the limits imposed by your fear of emotion.

Imagine if you could walk up to anyone without the fear that you had nothing interesting to say or that you would be unfavorably judged. Imagine if you could present your idea without caring what others thought. Imagine if you could be your authentic self without worrying about feedback from others? Imagine being able to do, be, or have whatever you want without the fear associated with failure. The thing you fear is the negative emotion. What if the negative emotion no longer caused pain? How would that change your life?

Negative emotion need not be painful when you see it as a message rather than a punishment. It's no longer painful when you can analyze it and release it rather than hang onto it. Negative emotion is no longer limiting when you can dismiss it quickly by choosing the proper perspective. When negative emotion no longer reigns over your life, your life expands dramatically.

If you are overweight, it's because you are having some difficulty managing your emotions. If you are drinking, smoking, or into some other substance that soothes you, it's because you have not learned how to deal with negative emotion. If you feel stress in your life, it's due to your inability to handle negative emotion. Your approach to life is simply not working. The way you are choosing to operate conflicts with what you want, what you intended to explore, and who you really are. You simply cannot continue to approach life in this manner. It's just not working and it never will.

You see the futility in believing that you are a victim of fate rather than the creator of your reality. You may see yourself as a creator, however, if you are approaching life from a standpoint of reaction instead of being proactive, you are operating in a broken system. You can't have it both ways. Either you are the creator or you are the victim. If you react like a victim, you're operating as a victim. If you want to be a creator, you must integrate the whole system. You must proactively choose your perspective. You must know what is really happening. You must understand that everything happens for you, not to you. You must give up your irrational fear of your own emotional guidance system. You must lean into life, not protect yourself from it. You must strive to accept your negative emotions and use them to your advantage. Anytime you feel negative emotion, it is a gift. If you can come to realize this one fact of reality, your life will dramatically improve in all areas.

IV.

Can you imagine accepting negative emotion as a gift? It seems impossible, doesn't it? How can you become so aware of yourself, of the world around you, and of your own fears and insecurities that you actually feel good when you receive negative emotion? It's all in your expectations, your attitude, and your approach to life.

You have created a habit of reaction. When something occurs that pleases you, you react favorably and you feel good. You adopt the higher perspective quite easily. You laugh, you giggle, you smile, and you enjoy the moment. The reaction is fully aligned with who you really are and what you really want. However, it is still a reaction.

When something happens and you react as if it were bad, without really thinking it through, you are immediately alerted to this limited perspective you've chosen. You feel bad. The feeling comes as a warning: "Do not look at this subject from the perspective that you've chosen." The perspective that you have decided to adopt will not serve you. It is a perspective that is limiting. It is a perspective that will cause you to attract that which we know you do not want. Drop this perspective quickly so that momentum does not build. Find a higher perspective. Look at the event or the subject again. Find a way to process this so that it serves what you want and who you are. Keep searching for a higher perspective until you feel relief. Once you've felt relief, you've found a better perspective. Once you feel joy, you've found the highest perspective.

Have you ever witnessed an event or even a story and felt goosebumps? This is a very high-vibrational feeling. It too is a message from your inner self. It lets you know that the perspective you've chosen on this subject perfectly aligns with who you really are and all that you truly want. The event that you are witnessing is happening for you. It's reinforcing some very beneficial beliefs. And the way you are choosing to see it is a most empowering perspective.

Positive emotion is a gift. It lets you know when you're on the right track. Along with the good feeling can come the knowledge that you are moving along just as you had intended and if you can keep this up, you'll receive all that you want.

Negative emotion is a gift too. But you don't yet realize this. Negative emotion helps you stay on track if you will only see the message. If you could get past your preoccupation with the feeling itself and analyze why you feel this way and deal with the underlying fear, you would return to feeling good so much faster. Instead, for some odd reason, you fight with the message contained in the emotion and you find a million reasons to hang onto your limited perspective.

It seems as if you want to justify your perspective. You believe your perspective is accurate. But if it does not serve you, what good is having an accurate perspective? If you know something to be true (which you cannot know, because nothing is that black or white) and that truth does not serve who you really are or help you move in the direction of what you want, then what difference does it make? Why make it such a big deal? If you are feeling negative emotion, it is because you are holding onto a perspective that is not true for you and you can release it. It is that simple.

Let's look at our previous example of a childhood within a ruined marriage. If you choose to look at it from a perspective that your parents' marriage failed, you are choosing a limited perspective. If you can find a higher perspective, such as "The marriage ran its course and this was part of the trajectory I chose," you have found an empowering perspective if it brings a feeling of relief. If you look back and say to yourself, "I see now that their divorce led me to believe this and that and those beliefs caused me to create this desire, which is what I really wanted after all. So now I see that the divorce led to some of the wonderful aspects of the life I now live."

If you feel relief, you've found an empowering perspective, and the emotional weight of the divorce will be a little lighter. If you can continue to find examples and proof that the divorce actually benefited you after all, you will release the negative emotion created by this event and your vibration will shift quite dramatically. When your vibration shifts in such a manner, your life moves to a new level. Your vibration attracts things that match it. When you release a limiting belief based in a strong fear, your life improves because your vibration no longer calls out looking for a match to this belief.

All limiting beliefs based in irrational fear are false. When you choose to believe that a limiting belief is a fact, or true, you are simply making that choice. It is always your choice. People may agree or disagree with your choice. People may think it is smart to hold onto or discuss their limiting beliefs, but it is not. It is simply limiting. You came here to live an unlimited life. You have total and complete freedom to choose your thoughts and your beliefs. The fact that you can choose your thoughts is proof that your life is designed to be limitless.

However, you choose to think limiting thoughts. You make the choice, not anyone else. No one tells you what to think; you allow or resist all thought. You choose to adopt or release your beliefs. You can reduce or increase the intensity of any belief. No one can tell you what to believe. It is all up to you.

Have you ever thought about why you chose to adopt a limiting belief? Because you did not understand what you were doing when it was happening. When you were a small child, you adopted all sorts of limiting beliefs that were given to you by those around you. You accepted their beliefs because you were told that they were smarter than you for the simple reason that they had lived longer than you and they presumed to know more. Their experience taught them certain things and you were told to believe them. And you did for the most part. You even adopted some of the crazier things they believed.

If you knew then what you know now, you would have taken their beliefs with a grain of salt. Their limiting beliefs may have been valid for them, but they did not apply to you. If you understood how the universe worked, you would not come to irrationally fear so many things. If you knew then that each person received that which they were a match to, you would simply focus on that which you wanted and ignore their limiting ideas and conversation.

If you have come to understand the basic fundamentals of the Law of Attraction, you already realize that you must take into account the vibrational impact of your thoughts, beliefs, words, and actions. When you express out loud that something is wrong, bad, or dangerous, you are simply adding that vibration to your own. Why would you want to bring in something that affects your vibration in a way that causes you to attract that which is not wanted? You would not, but you do it anyway. You think it doesn't matter, but it does.

Even the tiniest vibration of something you consider mildly bad or wrong affects your vibration. Imagine cooking a soup. You stir in all the ingredients and let it simmer. Soon they come together to create a wonderful flavor. Now you see a bottle of vinegar, which you do not like, but for some reason you decide to add it to your soup. Not much, just a few drops. How does the soup taste now? It's a different flavor, isn't it? It's not a bad flavor, it's just one you do not like. We are not saying it's bad or wrong to pay attention to things you do not prefer; we are only saying that you're adding something to the mix that is out of alignment with what you want. You're cooking a different kind of soup. It's not a bad soup; it's just one you do not prefer.

V.

If you do not like the feel, weight, or appearance of your body, it's because you are not consciously creating the body you desire. You are allowing your reaction to life to dictate how your body looks, how much money is in your bank account, who's lying in the bed next to you, and every other facet of your life. Nothing random is happening. It's all a reflection of your vibration brought forth into your personal reality. If you want it to improve, you must simply start focusing on what is wanted and remove your attention from what is not wanted.

This concept is very difficult for many people to understand. You have strong feelings about the things you do not like. You have a highly tuned habit of judgment. Your conversation primarily revolves around things you know you don't like. You have a limiting belief that you should voice your opinions, positive and negative. But this approach yields results that you do not want.

The first step in an approach to life that works within the laws of the universe is to start talking about things that are wanted. Start talking about things of great interest. Start thinking about new and positive ideas. Start asking to be guided toward conversations, thoughts, and ideas that are pleasing to you. Start intending to find people and conversations that revolve around the things you like.

In order to slow the momentum of the unwanted, it is important to refrain from speaking about the things you think are bad, wrong, or broken. Remove your attention from them. Stop believing they are bad or wrong. Start seeing some positive aspects of these things. Change your perspective on the subject. Disengage with those who want to talk about things they believe are wrong. Change the conversation or leave the room.

If you are unable to change the conversation and bring it around to things that are good and right with the world, then you must consider leaving the room. The art of changing the topic involves some level of confidence and tact. If you are insecure in your abilities, it is best to leave the room and escape the dialogue, because it does not serve you. Certainly, there is little point in watching the news or reading the newspaper. These things contain mostly gratuitous descriptions of events that do not require your attention.

In these modern times it is so easy to subscribe to blogs, podcasts, and news feeds that contain inspirational information and conversations that revolve around things that are of interest to you. You do not gain by reading about the most recent political scandal or about the ongoing war on this or that. It does not serve you. It is not empowering or inspirational. It is limiting.

The most common limiting habit is that of complaining. Complaining is powerful focus on that which you think is wrong. You believe that something that has already happened should be different than it is. If you think the conditions in the moment are less than perfect and you wish they would be different, you are reacting from an old paradigm that does not help you in any way. Complaining creates powerful momentum. That which you complain about gets worse, not better. You might think you are doing something to improve the situation when you complain, but all you are actually doing is causing the aspect you do not like to grow bigger and more distasteful.

This is an absolute fundamental element of the universe. You cannot escape it. If you think something is wrong or bad, you attract the negative aspects of it and add it to your vibration. If you decide to complain about something, your spoken words are powerful and you create an environment where the subject of your complaint becomes more pronounced and impactful. If you decide to take action against something you think is wrong, you create a monster out of it.

If you look at any action taken to irradiate a problem, you can see that the problem only gets worse. Look at the war on drugs. Those who decided that it was harmful for consenting adults to use drugs just made the entire subject worse by an order of magnitude. Now you have the highest prison population in the civilized world. Mexico has been decimated by this war. Countless lives have been squandered in the pursuit of this policy. Money has been diverted from areas where it could be beneficial and instead was used to keep this war funded. The fight against the problem causes the problem to exacerbate. When your government realizes that there never was a problem, simply the fear of a problem, they will work within the laws of the universe to create an environment they prefer. Fighting against a condition you believe is wrong only increases the perception of wrongness.

If you feel negative emotion in any conversation, you are adding something to your vibration that you do not want. It is best to stop the conversation then and there. When you practice this fine art of changing the subject, you'll get better and better at it. You will feel the slightest bit of negative emotion and this will alert you. You will know that the topic has gone into an area that is better left ignored. Those around you will still feel the urge to talk about things that are not in line with what you (or they) want. When you keep changing the conversation, they will start to pick up on what you're doing, and some will appreciate it and some will not. That's okay. It is better for you if you can control the topic of conversation and keep it centered on things that are interesting and pleasing. You are doing yourself a service as well as serving them in return.

When people spend enough time around you focusing more on what feels good and less on what is titillating or distressing, they will begin to feel better as well. Some will gravitate to you. Some seek higher-quality conversations. Some people are tired of the small talk and the petty conversations. However, there will always be those who are not vibrationally ready or able to maintain their focus on what's wanted. This requires a higher than average vibration and some are just not there yet. That is alright as well.

They will see your example and might one day be inspired by it. It might cause them to think about things in a new way. You cannot worry about other people in your life. They are on their own path. They are now and will always be at a different vibrational level than you. No one is at the same vibrational level at the same time. Allow them to stay in conversation with you if they can. If they cannot maintain this level of conversation, they will find someone else. It is important for you to keep up your standards and not to allow yourself to dip into lower-vibrational topics just to make others feel better or to appease them.

Your words are powerful. Use them with thought and intention. Intend to discuss topics of interest and inspiration. Intend to speak eloquently about things you like. Intend to remove yourself from any subject that is not appealing to you. Intend to remove your attention from unwanted things, even if you're a little curious. Realize that you do not need to be informed about anything that is not vibrationally uplifting. Focus on whatever you think is positive and remove your attention from whatever you personally view as negative.

One important thing to remember is that you have no control over what anyone else says, thinks, or does. If someone in your presence is talking about something that does not appeal to you, don't ask them to change. Don't make them wrong. Simply move the conversation to another topic. They will get it when you apply a little tact. However, if you attempt to make them wrong, they will simply dig in their heels and try to prove that they are right. You just can't win that battle.

VI.

By changing your approach to life, you are sending a signal to the universe that you are now choosing to consciously create the life you prefer. This is an excellent start. For the first few months, you'll be proactively choosing how you focus your attention on the things you like. You will try to control your thoughts. You might keep a journal of things you appreciate. You will be thinking about your conversations. You will be more tuned to your emotions. You will be noticing when things manifest. You will be realizing just how you are creating the conditions of your life.

You will also tend to look back at your past with regret and resentment. If you think of something you could have done differently, you might feel regret. If you look to a past event and believe others could have made better choices, you are feeling resentment. These negative emotions are indications that your perspective is off. When you look back into your past and blame yourself or others for the way things are now, you are using a very limited perspective and this is creating some of the things in your life that you want to be rid of. By looking at your past from the perspective of a victim, you are creating a future reality that perfectly aligns with that perspective.

But you say that the past is the past and there's nothing you can do about it. You're just facing reality. We disagree with that premise. The past is nothing more than your version of it. Your version comes from a very limited perspective. You can't know what led up to any event. You can't possibly know what others were feeling or dealing with. You only remember a few foggy pieces out of a huge, complex puzzle. The only thing you need to know is that the past unfolded perfectly to bring you to this exact point in time. If things didn't happen just as they did, you would not be here now. You are the highest version of you that has ever existed.

Everything did work out. You have never been at a higher vibration than you are now. You are finally ready to receive all that you want. You have finally made it to this place, which is the perfect place to start. You have finally made it to this level of vibration that allows you to understand what we are saying. That is a very high place indeed, because these concepts are not available to most people.

As you transition from a victim mentality to a creator mentality, you are really moving from irresponsibility to full responsibility. In the old approach, other things outside yourself had a lot to do with what happened. In this new approach, you are responsible for everything that happens in your world. You are now the center of your universe. You now control every single little thing that presents itself in your reality. All the people you know and the conditions that surround you are your responsibility. How they act is up to you. You create it all.

This is not an easy concept for most. If someone is rude to you, you believe that is their issue and has nothing to do with you. It might be their issue, but you are a vibrational match to it. If you were not, they could not show up in your reality. It simply isn't possible. If you get the first parking spot or find a quarter on the floor, you did that. You create all the good that comes into your life. You are also a vibrational match to anything that you perceive as negative as it enters your reality. You are a vibrational match to all of it. Isn't that good to know?

If someone is angry with you, you certainly created it. Are they being ridiculous? Only from your perspective. However, if it comes up, you have something to do with it. You are bringing it forth. It may have been waiting for you for a long time and now it's finally here. Your past approach to life created it and now you have to deal with it in your new approach. This is not so easy, but at least you can become aware of what's happening.

Let's say someone is angry with you for something you did not do. You think they are being completely unreasonable, yet if you were not a match to the qualities they are expressing, then it does match who you were being. That's okay. You don't need to fight it. You don't need to prove them wrong. You don't need to defend yourself. This is coming from your old way of being. You did not know what you were doing; it stemmed from your unconscious approach to life. Now you are thinking more. Now you are choosing your words. Now you are intending to do that which aligns with what you want and who you really are. Your new approach to life is filled with conscious choices, while your old approach to life was based on unconscious reactions. There is a huge difference between the two.

When you simply reacted unconsciously to the events in the outside world, you created unconsciously and you received some of what you wanted and some of what you did not want. You developed a persona and your ego fought to preserve the dignity of this fabricated version of yourself. That's okay. However, things have changed. You know more now. You are moving to a new way of living. You are intending to experience a higher-quality life. You are now choosing to react to the conditions in a brand new way. You are now consciously choosing your reactions.

Can you see how a defensive reaction to life could create a life that allows in things you do not want? If something happens and you judge it to be bad, you are placing your attention on the aspects of the event that you do not like and you're adding that to or keeping that in your vibration. You aren't getting anywhere. You are not progressing as you would like. Some things you judge as good and some things you judge as bad and so you have a vibration that contains a relatively even mix of good and bad. This is unconscious creation. You are still creating by your focus of attention; it's just that you're not aware of the ramifications of your focus.

Now imagine what a conscious creator looks like. You are still reacting happily to things that are good, but now you are removing your attention from things you do not like. It's your attention that creates your reality. When you look at something and think it's wrong, you are paying attention to it and adding it to your vibration. You are creating by looking at it. You are adding it to your soup and your soup is your creation, because this soup is all you have.

In this new and powerful approach to life, you have the conscious ability to be, do, and have anything you like. What you receive is a match to how you feel. If you feel good, good-feeling things will waltz into your life. This approach to life centers around feeling good, feeling confident, having faith, and choosing an empowering perspective. This is an approach to life where you intend to create what is wanted by learning to maintain high-flying, positive feelings as much as humanly possible. For the first time in your life, you are going to really understand the simple fact that you are the center of your universe, you come first, and you create your personal reality. It is all up to you. It always has been and it always will be. You are more powerful than you can imagine. Now let's show you how to wield that power

Chapter Seven

Learning to Leverage Universal Forces to Create the Life You Want

There are universal laws, such as the Law of Attraction. This law says that what you put forth is returned to you. You attract those things into your reality that are a match to your vibration. It's one thing to understand the idea; it's another thing to put it into practice on a daily basis. Learning to live within the laws of the universe is the new approach to life we are suggesting. Some people are able to do this instinctively without knowing anything about these laws, but most people are living in a way that fights against universal laws.

You can easily spot the people who naturally abide by the laws of the universe. They are happy, positive, easygoing, and seem to go with the flow of life. They are optimists. They are confident. They love themselves and others. They see the good and do not spend much time on things they do not like. You might call them Pollyanna, yet this is the approach to life that naturally aligns with the forces of the universe.

Universal forces are quite powerful. These same forces created worlds, stars, and galaxies. If these forces can create galactic wonders, imagine the power they can wield in your life. When you learn to use universal forces to your benefit, things happen easily. When you live in opposition to these laws, everything is harder. Your approach to life determines how these forces work for you or against you. Again, it is all up to you.

Imagine a life where you are completely cared for, loved, and supported from cradle to grave. Everything is provided for you. You can be, do, and have anything you want simply by asking for it. You can explore any aspect of physical reality you choose. Imagine having the ability to bring anything into your life simply by altering your vibration. This is the reality that exists for you now. This is the reality that has always existed for you. This is the design and purpose of this reality. This is the reason you chose to come here.

Now imagine that you were taught a different reality. You were taught that you can't have anything you want. You were taught not to be selfish. You were programmed to believe you were not safe and that you had to defend yourself against all dangers, real and perceived. You were taught that others controlled your fate and that you were either lucky or unlucky. These ideas, which go against the actual reality of this system, caused you to approach life in a way that simply could not work. Since much of your reality is determined by your beliefs, your reality matches what you believe. When that happens, the illusion becomes so strong and ingrained, it's hard to break away from it.

Then we come along to teach you about a new reality. What we say makes sense and you resonate with much of it because it sounds familiar. There is truth in what we say, even when your beliefs are telling you otherwise. It's not that you're learning anything new; it feels more like you are remembering what you once knew. This is because you are a vibrational match to this information. If you were not a match to it, you could not be reading this book right now. Somehow, in the midst of many limiting beliefs, your vibration held the key that was necessary to unlock this information. This is how the universe works.

There are many universal laws and principles that are in conflict with some of your tightly held, limiting beliefs. In order for you to come around to actually consciously creating your life on purpose, you must reduce the intensity of these beliefs and learn to work with the universal principles. This takes time. It will seem difficult. It will take patience and practice, but it will be well worth it.

Before we begin, let's recap some of the universal principals that you must realize to be true for you before you can integrate this higher approach to life.

You are worthy. You are as worthy as any who have ever lived and as worthy as any who will ever step foot on Planet Earth. Can you really come to believe that statement? It is absolutely true. You are part of One. All parts of One are equal. You came here to experience life in a way that has never been experienced before and will never be experienced again. All experiences are equally valid. The experience of the homeless man is just as valid, important, and relevant as the life experience of your president. One is not higher or better than the other in universal terms. They are equal. You might judge one to be preferable or even more important, but it is not. It is simply your way of processing the information. Your perspective causes you to seek definitions and judgments that create hierarchies. In universal terms, there are no levels of importance. It is all equally important.

You are unique. No one looks like you, acts like you, thinks like you, or has the same special gifts as you do. No one ever has or ever will be anything like you. Your gifts are important to the expansion of the universe. Imagine you are a superhero with unique talents. Each superhero has their strengths and each can do something the other cannot. Have you found your superpowers yet? If not, it's probably because you don't consider them to be anything special. You tend to compare yourself to others and wish you had their talents and gifts. But for you, your powers are very special and you specifically chose them prior to your entry into physical reality.

You have full access to well-being. Everything you need is being provided to you not by your own efforts or by anyone else, but by the power and the energy of the universe. You are being fed energy at all times by the universe. You can feel the energy or the lack of it. When you feel great, you feel the energy and when you feel terrible, you feel the lack of it. It does not come to you from outside sources. There is no one sending you energy. You are not plugged into a wall; it comes from the universe. It comes from the inside. It comes from Source.

You can choose to allow the energy to flow, but you cannot force it to flow. You can cut off the energy if you wish. You decide what to think and where to place your focus and this determines whether you are allowing energy to come or whether you are temporarily cutting it off or resisting it in some way. If you relax and allow it to flow, it flows. If you are resistant to the conditions that surround you because you perceive them to be bad or wrong, you might restrict that flow unintentionally.

Everything is right. There is no wrong anywhere in the universe. If you choose to see something as bad or wrong, you are simply resisting it. It is right. You can choose a perspective that aligns with who you are and what you want and see the subject of your focus as right, or you can choose the perspective that makes it wrong. Either way, it's your choice. The subject is actually neutral and your judgment makes it right or wrong. When it's right to you, you are allowing the energy to flow and you are working with the forces of the universe. When you see it as wrong, you are fighting against universal forces and you are limiting the energy and well-being that can flow to you.

You have a guidance system. You have an inner self who is you as you still exist in the nonphysical. Your inner self knows every thought you think, what you truly want, and who you really are. Your inner self sees everything from the higher perspective. Your inner self knows how to get you where you want to go, even though you can't see it. Your inner self becomes a vibrational match to whatever you want and creates a pathway and a process for you to become a match as well.

If you feel negative or positive emotion of any strength, this is a message from your inner self. When the emotion feels bad, the message says "choose a new perspective. The way you're looking at this subject is out of alignment with what you want. You are moving in the wrong direction. You are stepping off the path." Change your perspective or use the art of analysis until you feel relief. Once you feel better, this feeling is your indication that you've gotten back on track.

When you feel positive emotion, it is also a message from your inner self. It is letting you know that how you are looking at the subject is in perfect alignment with your desires. You are on track and you're moving closer to becoming a vibrational match to that which you desire. Revel in these moments and realize that this love energy is supporting you every step of the way. Realize that your perspective is right on target. Get really good at choosing the aligned perspective.

Guidance also comes in the form of intuition and direct communication. When you are feeling good, you'll receive inspiration to act. In these moments, act. Do not doubt, just perform the action that you are thinking about. As long as you are in a higher emotional state of being and you take action that comes from inspiration, the action will always create a result that is necessary for your growth and expansion. It may not always seem like it at the time, but the action is part of the process that will modify your vibration and transform you into the version of you that is ready for what you want to manifest into your reality.

Demand to feel good. This is a feeling reality and all that ever matters is how you feel. When you feel good, you have full access to universal forces, source energy, and abundance and well-being. When you feel good, you are allowing the energy to flow. You are in the state of allowing. You are creating an environment where everything you want is coming to you. You create what is wanted by feeling good first, not by coercing the conditions in a way that allows you to feel good. Feel good in spite of the conditions and the conditions will improve. When you ask the conditions or the people in your life to be different than they are, just to make you feel better, you are fighting against the conditions. This approach does not work.

Allow the conditions and the people in your life to be just as they are. Accept them for who and what they are. Change your perspective so that you may feel better, but do not ask them to change for you. They might try to change for you and this approach may seem efficient and effective, but they can never be who you want them to be all of the time. When they go back to being who they are, and you get annoyed by this, you will return to feeling bad.

Learn to feel good. Learn to allow everything to be good as it is without requiring it to be different in the moment. Seek out the positive aspects of everything and focus on them. If you can keep yourself feeling good, your reality will improve to match your feelings. It is law and cannot be any other way. The art of feeling good in the face of any and all conditions also takes some practice and commitment. Your current approach to life does not require you to feel good. Feeling good is not something you strive for. In your current approach to life you seek out situations and conditions that will hopefully cause you to feel good, but you never know. You want to react to the conditions around you and feel good as a side effect. However, in this new approach to life, you will be asked to feel good first and then watch as the universe responds with many good-feeling moments.

Can you see how your current approach to life is backwards? You enter a condition and your reaction to that condition causes you to feel good or bad. It's the condition that causes the response. You have little control over your feelings, so you choose conditions that have the potential to make you react positively. If the condition isn't good, or if you cannot respond positively to the condition, you feel bad. You are trying to avoid feeling bad by creating conditions that cause you to feel good. But this is a haphazard approach to life.

Let's present an example.

You like to fish. You think that fishing is fun. You buy a boat, buy the gear, buy bait, fuel, food, and drinks, get your friends together, and go fishing. Why do you do this? Because you think it will be fun and fun feels good. You do all of this hoping to feel good. But will you actually feel good? Maybe yes and maybe no. If everything goes according to plan, your reaction will be to feel good. If the weather is nice, if the fish are biting, if the beer is cold, if the boat works, if you have enough money, if your friends are in a good mood, if no one gets hurt, if everything lines up perfectly, then and only then will you feel good. That's a lot of ifs. You are counting on a lot of variables to go your way just to feel good.

Here's the funny thing. None of it will go well if you don't already feel good. If you feel good first, then things will line up. But, if you feel bad, then things will work out to match how you are feeling. If you wake up and the weather is overcast, this might set you off on a bad emotional state of being. You might be disappointed. If you are short on money but have to buy all the gas, food, and drinks, this might create a sour mood that will affect the rest of the day.

You create from the inside out, not the outside in. You feel something and the world around you lines up with that feeling. The feeling always comes first. The reason fishing is either fun for you or not fun is because of how you feel. If you like fishing, fishing is generally fun, because you've had fun times in the past and that momentum carries forth. You have positive expectations and those expectations create a fun day fishing. If you don't like fishing it's because you have had a previous set of experiences in which fishing did not create good feelings. You think the experience creates the feeling, so if an experience is pleasing, you like it and if it's not, you don't. It's not the experience itself — it's you. It's always you.

Your emotional state of being has a lot to do with what you create. If you can feel good and maintain a high emotional state of being, you will receive experiences and conditions that match how you feel. If you feel good, you will receive things that match that. You will receive inspiration to do or not do something. If you desire a lean and healthy body, you will receive inspiration that aligns with this desire. You might be inspired to drink water, to exercise, to find healthy recipes, or to read certain books that will have an impact on your beliefs. Whatever the inspiration is, it will be specific to you. You will like it and want to do it. It will be enjoyable.

If you are in a low emotional state of being, you will also receive inspiration in the form of urges. However, the inspiration will match your state of being. It will inspire you to do something to relieve your bad feelings. You might be inspired to gossip, smoke a cigarette, have a drink, or eat a tub of ice cream. The inspiration in this case is designed to improve your feelings, not to help you achieve your desire. In fact, the urge might be at odds with your desire.

This causes emotional conflict. Imagine you want to lose weight, but you find yourself in a low emotional state of being because you don't like the shape of your body. Your inspiration is to soothe yourself by eating. This temporarily feels good, but since it is in conflict with your desire, you feel bad. Momentum is created and it feels like you cannot get out of this rut. It all has to do with how you are feeling.

Feel good first and everything you want will flow to you. Feel bad, and you limit what can come to you. Create from the inside by feeling good and allowing good-feeling things to come. Do not ask the conditions to change shape just to please you. Be pleased by whatever conditions exist and they will begin to improve. Accept everything as right and you enter the state of allowing. It is from this position that you will receive that which you want, including a lean body.

II.

This reality is designed to bring you everything you want, yet you persist in your resistance. You believe that you know how things should unfold, so you try to coerce the conditions to get what you want. You effort your way to what you think you want. But effort is doing things without the leverage of universal forces. When you take some form of action on your own to create what you think you want, you go it alone. The universe is not working with you when you take matters into your own hands. In order to be truly powerful in this reality, you must align yourself with the powers of the universe.

You do not really understand what you want when you ask for something. Therefore, you can never really know how to go out and get it. What you really want is the feeling something will bring, not the thing itself. If you want a vacation and you imagine a beach on a tropical island, you may really want time away from work, a reduction in stress, to spend some time alone with your mate, an adventure, or any number of things. When you imagine the feeling of what you want, you create a mental picture. You are only able to imagine what you have already seen in movies, magazines, photos, or past experiences. You are not really able to imagine something more than that. However, the universe always knows how to bring you the most exciting and elegant manifestation of your desire. You can't even begin to imagine what the universe can do.

You want the feeling of these things and the universe knows how to create a reality that perfectly matches or exceeds the feelings you desire. When you think you have to make it happen on your own, you create something far less magical and ultimately unsatisfying. You will put yourself in the situation, but you don't receive the feeling you imagined and you're disappointed.

Can you look back at a time in your life when you planned something out but it didn't turn out to be as satisfying as you imagined? You made the effort to create something, maybe a trip or maybe the manifestation of a thing, and it just didn't feel like you thought it would. We see this happening all too frequently. Now think back to something you wanted that you received without much, if any, planning. Think about a time when you just went with the flow and everything worked out magically. When you try to create something yourself, you are fighting against the flow of life. When you allow the universe to work it out for you, you are going with the flow of life.

There is a flow to life and when you relinquish your control, magical things will start happening for you. You do not have to fight this flow; you can simply allow yourself to move in unison with it. The universe knows what you truly want and how to get it. It sends you signals when it's time to act. These signals feel like ideas, thoughts, inspiration, and intuition. It feels right. It feels fun. You want to do it. It seems logical. When you act from inspiration, you are leveraging the forces of the universe and you become highly effective at manifesting that which you desire.

Doesn't this make sense to you? If this reality is designed to bring you what you want, why would you have to do anything other than that which is done out of inspiration? If this reality is creating manifestations for you, the only time you would need to take any action is when things are perfectly lined up.

Imagine you were orchestrating a manifestation. Let's say you are your inner self. You know what your physical self wants, what you're thinking, and what your vibration is emitting. You know all the beliefs and fears that are attached to your physical self. You can see everything from the higher perspective. You know what to do and how to make it all come together to bring your physical self the feelings it really wants to experience.

You, as your own inner self, know how the universe works. You are intimately familiar with the laws of the universe and you know how to leverage universal forces. You know what you intended to explore prior to your physical self's birth. You know how worthy and unique your physical self is and you are eager to guide the physical you toward that which you are here to explore. Knowing all this, what would you do?

You know the complete and total desire that the physical you has created. You understand the true essence of this desire and the feeling of it. It doesn't matter what the desire is; as the inner self, you have no judgment one way or the other. If your physical self has birthed a desire, you are there to bring it forth into reality.

The first place you will start is by working on your physical self's vibration. The vibration is not aligned with the desire because there are a few limiting beliefs standing in the way. You must create manifestation events that will alert your physical self to the fear at the basis of these beliefs. So you set up the conditions and you work with other inner selves to create these important events. When the time is right, you will send your physical self inspiration to act. If your physical self goes with the inspiration, the manifestation event will occur. If not, you'll try again. You'll never stop creating manifestation events in an effort to modify your physical self's vibration so that it might become vibrationally aligned with its desire.

From the higher perspective, you can see the landscape so much better. You know who needs to be involved, where to go, what to look for, what action needs to take place, and, most importantly, the timing of everything. From the limited perspective of your physical self, you can't see any of this, yet you think you can. Imagine being in a corn maze on a sunny day. You enter the maze and you just keep turning corners and trying to remember where you are. You keep getting stuck in lanes that lead to dead ends. You can only see the next corner in front of you and you have to remember where you've been. You have to backtrack and try one route after another until you finally make it to the other side and find the exit. However, if you could see the maze from the higher perspective, say forty feet above the maze, you could find your way out of the maze quickly and easily.

We hear you say that the maze is designed to be fun and challenging and we get your point. You want to be challenged and you like the feeling of success. That is all well and good. But if you are in the maze and you're constantly running into the same dead ends, wouldn't it be nice to hear a little voice whisper "This way" once in a while? That is what your inner self is doing when you feel inspiration.

There is no rush to achieve your dreams. Most of the fun is on the journey as your dream unfolds. It's just that your inner self is part of that journey. You came here knowing you would receive guidance along the way. You never intended to go it alone. It is not more satisfying doing it by yourself. You wanted to create your desires in alignment with your inner self and the powers of the universe. You wanted to do it together. You came here to become a master of creation and you create by aligning with the forces of the universe and through the guidance received from your inner self.

III.

How do you create anything you desire? By creating a vibration that is in harmony with the desire. How do you adjust your vibration so that it comes into the same frequency as your desire? By allowing the universe to do it for you. The universe brings your desire to you. The universe lines everything up. The universe works to change your vibration so that it matches your desire. The universe causes you to feel the inspiration to act. Your guidance system lets you know when you are working with the universe and when you are not. It is an elegant system.

In the nonphysical, we create whatever it is we want from pure thought. We think of what is wanted and it appears. Do we think we created it? Of course. Did we actually do anything more than think the thought and fully expect the thought to manifest? No. That's all creation is. But how did the desire actually manifest? The universe made it happen.

When you turn on a light switch, did you actually turn on the lights? Of course you did. However, there is a power plant somewhere that is sending the energy through power lines and into your home. Did the power plant turn on your lights? No, you did. It just made it happen when you decided you wanted light. You did not create the power, you simply utilized it for lighting, or cooking, or television, or music, or any number of things. The power of the universe is very similar in that respect. You make the decision or birth the desire and the universe provides the power to make it happen.

When you take action thinking you are going to create the result through sheer effort and will power, you do not engage the power of the universe. Imagine wanting light in your house and instead of turning on the light by flicking a switch, you wad up an old newspaper and you light it on fire. Sure, there is some light, but it is not long-lasting, efficient, or useful. It is a paltry substitute for a lamp and electricity.

You have this power at your fingertips, but you might not have understood that it existed or how to engage it. Like electricity, the power is always on. You use switches to engage it, just as you use switches to engage the electricity in your home. You can leave the lights on or turn them off. It is the switch that holds back the power or allows it to flow.

When you feel good, the switch is on and the power flows. When you do not feel good, you either restrict the power (like a dimmer switch) or you turn it off. It's never completely off, but you understand the analogy we are making. We will say that when you are in a state of despair, the switch is almost off and when you are in any other negative state of being, the switch is dimmed to a degree that corresponds with your level of emotional distress. If you feel hatred, the power is dimmed substantially. If you feel bored, the power is dimmed just a little.

In order to efficiently manifest what you want, you must leave the switch all the way on as much as possible. The supply of universal energy is inexhaustible. You will never run out. There's no need to conserve it. Leave the switch on all the time. Let it flow continuously. You intended to live a life where you fully engaged the powers of the universe. You never intended to cut yourself off from the flow of energy for too long.

The flow of energy is constant. It comes from source energy directly to you. It does not waver; it is always there. The only possible way you could receive less energy is by cutting yourself off from it because you have chosen to see something as wrong and you've allowed that to determine the mood you will adopt. When you allow the conditions that exist in the outside world to influence you away from the energy stream, you restrict the flow of energy yourself. No one else is causing the flow to cease but you. You are in complete control of the energy stream. You either accept the full amount or you unconsciously choose to limit the flow. It's completely up to you.

The outside conditions are your personal creation. You created it all. You created the good and the bad. You created your definition of good and your description of bad. You created the perspective that can even tell the difference. Everything is neutral. You decide what is good or bad. Other people may offer their opinions, but ultimately, it is all up to you. You make the choice.

When you see something and place your judgment on it, you label it either good or bad or somewhere in the middle. It is not good or bad; it is neutral. So then, when you say that something is good or right, you are choosing to keep the power switch in the up position and you're allowing the flow to continue at its maximum rate. When you label it as bad or wrong, you are reducing the flow to a degree depending on how bad or wrong you think it is. Your judgment is the switch.

Judge something that you created (and you created everything and every person) as good, the switch is up. Judge it as bad or wrong and the switch is down. Up is fully engaged. Down is limiting.

Can you find a way to see something as good even when you believe it is wrong? Absolutely. The belief that it is wrong is limiting. It limits the flow of energy. It limits your experience of life. It limits your ability to manifest what you desire. It can be seen as good and right. You can flip the switch. You can reengage the energy. You can get things moving as soon as you can reduce the intensity of the limiting belief and see the subject as good and right. You don't have to shy away from the subject. There is a way to understand that it is good and right. Anything you currently believe to be wrong can be seen as right if you understand that there is no benefit to seeing it as wrong and great benefit in seeing it as right.

Imagine that you have an autistic child. Your child is not like other children; he has a unique set of attributes that make him different from those children you might label as normal. He is unique. If you believe that this condition is wrong, you will slip into a low emotional state of being and thereby cut yourself off from the energy stream. You will notice how he is different. You will want him to be something he is not. You might blame yourself or others for his condition. You might seek a treatment in the hopes that he may one day become normal. All of this restricts the flow of energy to you.

You can only allow or restrict the flow of energy to yourself. You cannot control the flow of others, but you can and do influence them to either restrict or allow their flow. If you see something as wrong and you get everyone else to see your point of view, you might cause them to restrict their own flow. If you inspire them to see the subject as perfectly good and fine, you might influence them to open their own flow.

If you believe that your child came here with the intention to view the world from a completely new and unique perspective and that he intended to live life in a way where others would have little influence on him and so he chose this condition intentionally for that reason, then you might allow yourself to feel better and the flow of energy is opened. If you could see that all children are unique and that there is no normal, you might open the flow. If you could see that there is no treatment needed and he is perfect as he is, then you open your flow.

You choose to restrict or open the flow. We ask you to keep your flow open.

IV.

There is a flow to life. The universe is constantly moving you in the direction toward what is wanted. You have a very limited point of view. From your perspective, you cannot see very far down the road. You cannot know what is being set up. You do not know how your beliefs must be changed. However, the universe knows it all. If you are to go with the flow of life, you must come to understand that everything is happening for you and nothing is happening to you.

This is a very important concept that you must come to grasp if you are to live a life of ease. The only way to go with the flow of life is to ease into it. When you think you must fight, struggle, and effort your way to what you want, you are not engaging the powers of the universe. When you believe that you must make it happen on your own, you are not going with the flow of life. It is supposed to be easy. When your life is not being easy, simply take a step back, give up your resistance, and allow the universe to take over.

There are many paths that will lead you to the manifestation of your desire and they are all downhill. Isn't that an interesting concept? Nothing you want is uphill. Nothing you want needs to be hard. You might work hard to prove you've sacrificed something in order to reach your goal, but this is simply a facet of your society. Your society favors hard work and sacrifice. In your society, these things are respected. You might believe that people simply do not respect those who receive things easily. Yet the ones who go with the flow of life and engage the forces of the universe are the ones who are playing the game effectively. They are doing the real work. The work is an inside job. The universe responds to this work by reflecting it on the outside world.

Give up your idea of effort and struggle. If it is difficult, if it is painful, if it is a struggle, then you are not engaging the forces of the universe and you're not going with the flow of life. If you are doing something you do not enjoy in the hope you will lose weight, you cannot create a lean body that will remain lean for very long.

Your effort may yield some temporary results, but unless you've engaged the forces of the universe and have done your inner work (reducing the intensity of limiting beliefs, altering your perspective, changing your approach to life, etc.), all your effort will be for naught. The changes will not stick. You might lose a few pounds for a few months, but the weight will gradually return.

You have seen examples of this many times. You get to a point where you do not like what you see in the mirror. This is contrast. You feel bad. You are having a manifestation event as you look in the mirror. So you decide to make a change. Generally, you want to remove yourself from the condition of having a fat body. You do not like the conditions as they are, so you decide to change the conditions. If you are looking at your own body in the mirror and you are judging it as bad or wrong, you are looking at an outside condition. When you seek to remove yourself from the condition, you are focusing all your attention on the condition. When you do this, the universe assumes that you are looking at something you like and it keeps you fat, or makes you fatter.

Have you ever been on a diet that did not work? It's because you were focused on a subject you did not like and the universe saw your point of focus and brought you more of that. You engaged the forces of the universe. They are very powerful forces. You did not engage them to move you to a new place; instead, you wanted to remove yourself from this place. Do you see the difference? When you desire to go to a new place, you aren't hating the existing place. In fact, you are appreciating the current place while looking forward in anticipation of your journey to the new place. This is how you leverage the powers of the universe. You work with them, not against them.

When you hate your body as it is, you are placing a lot of attention on what is and the universe responds to that attention. There is no good or bad in the universe; everything is neutral. The universe seeks to bring you that which you are paying attention to. It assumes that if you are focused on something, you must like that thing, otherwise you would focus your attention elsewhere. Doesn't that make sense? When you focus your attention on something you think is wrong, the universe brings more of that into your life.

How does the universe keep you fat? The ways are too numerous to count. It makes your cravings increase. It puts you in situations that tempt you. It brings you together with others who are going through the same issues with their bodies as you are. It will bring you articles, news stories, and conversations that confuse you and cause you to believe that what you're doing is ineffective. When you are focused on your body by thinking that it is not good as it is, the universe will bring you examples and put you in situations that reinforce this limiting belief. It's simply the Law of Attraction at work.

So how in the universe are you to move from where you are now to where you want to go? How are you to lose weight and keep it off? What are you going to do? Are you going to try another diet? Are you going to starve yourself? Are you going to buy some new exercise apparatus you've just seen on TV? No, because that is all working on the conditions you are observing on the outside. That is just trying to change your outer world. If you want to really change, you must change from the inside out.

When you change who you are, your outer world changes to match the inner you. The outer world, including your body, is a reflection of your inner world. When you seek to change your outer world, you might cause it to change a little, but if you have not changed your inner world, your outer world will gradually change back to reflect how you really feel on the inside. Isn't this good news?

The reason nothing has changed for you is because you haven't changed. Until you make some fundamental changes, your outer reality will not change. Nothing will change. However, once you make some small changes to who you are being right now, then everything changes. Not only will your body improve, but everything else will improve right along with it. Your relationships will improve, your finances will improve, your mood will improve, your health will improve. Everything gets better when you decide to become who you really are.

Chapter Eight

Change Made on the Inside Creates a New Reality on the Outside

In order for the conditions that surround you to change, you must change first.

For most people reading this book there is a belief that when the outside conditions change to please them, they will feel better. They believe that the conditions that appear in their physical reality cause them to feel either good or bad. So if they can control the conditions and keep the conditions nice enough, they will feel good most of the time. They are creating from the outside in.

By now you must know that this is the old approach to life, which simply does not work in this attractive reality. This environment was designed to be created by you based on what you wanted, how you felt, and what you paid attention to. You create from the inside out. However, when you react to the outside conditions first, you are allowing the conditions that exist to create your reality. This is why you may feel stuck or helpless. If you are most often reacting to the conditions with appreciation and joy, then your conditions will get even better. However, if you are reacting to the conditions of your life with disdain and anger, your conditions will change to increase these negative feelings. The conditions will get worse.

If you could change your approach to life to one where you seek to feel good and then allow the conditions to improve in response to how you are now feeling, your life experience would improve immensely. You create what you want by birthing a desire and focusing your attention on that desire while appreciating the life you have now, even though the thing you want is not yet in your life. Do you see the difference between this new approach and your old approach? In the old approach to life, you birthed a desire and then you complained that it had not yet arrived. You derided the conditions that existed before your desire was manifested and you felt like a victim. You believed that once the desire came, you'd be happy. Until then, you were content to be miserable. This approach goes against the laws of the universe and that's why it just cannot work and will never work.

No one has received their true desire by hating where they are while they were on the road to their desire. It could not happen, because it goes against the laws of the universe. If you believe there is an example of someone who became a success by hating where they came from, you cannot know the whole story. If someone did not like where they were and wanted to find a way out, the conditions may have appeared to change, but their inner feelings remained the same. There are countless examples of people who came from nothing and rose to great success, yet many of them never enjoyed that success because they could not escape the place they came from.

It's not the conditions on the outside that matter; it's always how you feel on the inside that is important. The conditions may change and to the outside observer, they may appear to be improved, but unless the person changes who they are on the inside, the conditions will still represent the same old feelings. The outside may look different, but it will always bring up the same feelings that are being felt on the inside.

Your outer reality is a representation of how you feel on the inside. If you feel bad on the inside, your conditions, no matter how they look, will continue to cause you to feel bad. They are simply and only a reflection of how you feel on the inside. That's it. You could make an effort and physically change the appearance of your outer conditions and for a while you might feel better. But the conditions are not creating a change within you; you are creating the change in your outside conditions and therefore no real inner change is taking place. Soon enough, when the illusion of change goes away, things will start to feel the way they always did and everything in your outer reality will feel a lot like it always did.

If you make real change on the inside, your reality will gradually (sometimes immediately) change to reflect the new you. Your conditions will begin to make you feel as good on the outside as you feel on the inside. Everything will start to make you happy. The outer world will present situations and examples that cause you to feel as good or even better than you feel on the inside. It's perfectly fine to react to good-feeling moments by feeling good and appreciating them. This reinforces your good feelings and you build momentum. How you react to the outside conditions paves the way for your future. If you react to the present moment in happiness and joy, your future will be more of this. If you react out of despair and frustration, you are more likely to receive a future that feels like that.

Change is not as difficult as it appears. You are constantly in a state of change. You are a fluid being, always and forever changing. You could not possibly be static for even a moment in time because with each new moment, you are forever changed. Every cell in your body is changing also. Millions of cells are dying and new ones are replacing them. Your body is in a constant state of flux. It is a completely new body every moment as it loses and receives cells. You cannot keep yourself from changing, so why not embrace change?

As you have heard many times before, change is the only constant. This is a very accurate statement. However, the change you create on the outside will not cause you to change who you are on the inside for very long.

Let's imagine you lose twenty pounds and you look and feel better than you have for years. You buy a new wardrobe and you get a new haircut. You look in the mirror and you like what you see. You believe the difficult diet and the painful exercise was all worth it. You feel really good. But why do you feel good? Is it a feeling of now being worthy? Do you feel pride in accomplishment? Do you feel attractive to others? What is it that changed?

There is a vibration that was being emitted from you that resonated with the feeling of being overweight. There's no need to dwell on the specific reason. There are many feelings that can lead to weight gain. One of them is insecurity about the worthiness of self. The feelings of unworthiness can lead to obesity, poverty, loss of freedom, physical or emotional abuse, failure, financial ruin, and many other unwanted conditions. Unless these feelings are resolved, the conditions will always revert to something unwanted that reinforces feelings of unworthiness.

Let's say you felt unworthy and you took a look at the conditions of your life and you created a desire to make a change. In this case, we will say that you felt unworthy and that these feelings manifested themselves as poverty. You look around and you see others who are successful and making money. You believe that if you could just get some money, you would alleviate your feelings of unworthiness. You become determined and you take a job you do not like, but you are driven by the conditions you hate. Soon enough you will have made some money and with the money you change the appearance of your conditions by renting a nice apartment and buying a new car.

But the conditions don't make you feel more worthy over the long run. The conditions can fool you into believing you are more worthy, but this won't last. You must feel worthy first. You must find a way to feel worthy and then allow the conditions to change on their own. Unless you find a way to feel more worthy, you will lose the car and the apartment and you might find yourself in conditions that feel even worse.

If you decide to change the shape of your body through starvation dieting and excessive exercise, you might make a change to the outside appearance of your body and you might feel better for a time, but if the core feelings don't change, you'll gain the weight back and feel even worse about yourself. This is why conventional diets don't work.

Typical diets all seek to change the outer conditions. If the inner feelings are not substantially changed, the outer conditions will always go back to how they were or even get worse. Long-term change must come from the inside. It is your feelings that create your reality.

You may know someone who is ultra-successful and confident, but overweight. How is this possible? Obviously, they must feel worthy, otherwise how would they be so successful? It's because they feel worthy in some areas of their life and unworthy in others. They are confident in some areas, yet insecure in others. Few people have consciously chosen to create an environment of worthiness in all facets of their lives and so some areas are more successful than others. There is nothing wrong with this; it is just due to their ignorance of the laws of the universe.

Your self-doubt, your worry, your insecurity and your feelings of unworthiness are all created by limiting beliefs about yourself and they are simply not true. In this moment in time you stand on the precipice of a great and wonderful future. If you are reading this book now, your vibration is a match to this information. You are at a very high vibrational level. If you can understand our words, you can improve how you feel on the inside and then allow your world to change on the outside.

There is no trick to change. It is not difficult, but it takes a little belief, a little patience, and a little practice. You are able to consciously create a future where your body is lean and feels good to you, where your relationships are strong and love surrounds you, and where all of your dreams are manifesting all around you. If you believe that you can change how you feel about yourself, then that is all that is required. We will show you the way.

II.

You are not being asked to change who you are; we are asking you to become who you really are. You are a being of pure positive love and acceptance. Who you really are is one who loves those in your life unconditionally and who accepts the conditions as they are. That's who you really are. If you are behaving in a way that is less than this, you are simply pretending to be someone you are not.

You were born into this world with the intention of living a life of joy, freedom, ease, abundance, expansion, and exploration. If your life is not like this now, you are acting in a way that is out of alignment with how you intended to live. It is really quite a lot more difficult to be who you are not than who you really are. It is difficult to pretend to be someone else.

You came to this world wanting to explore certain aspects of reality and so you chose your parents, the time and place of your birth, and your specific body with all its unique features and attributes. You knew that the environment of your youth would launch you on a trajectory toward where you wanted to go and what you wanted to explore. You chose it all. You chose your unique gifts and talents. You like who you really are, but you may fear showing this to others.

Fear is what keeps you from expressing who you really are. You want to fit in. You want to be accepted. You want to be loved. So you try to diminish the outstanding and unique qualities of yourself in fear of standing out and being different. Let's face it together. You are different. You are unique. You do have special gifts and talents and a unique personality. You have a truly unique outlook on life. You have a perspective that has never existed in the history of the world and will never exist again. You are special, unique, worthy, and important. Your life adds to the expansion of the universe. Without you, the universe would be less than it is now.

When you change who you are being now to become who you really are, you will find success in all areas of your life. When you are being who you really are, you fully engage the powers of the universe and you are aligned with everything you want. When you suppress who you are out of fear, you disengage some or all of the powers of the universe and you can't really accomplish anything of substance.

When you are limiting who you are out of fear, you are really avoiding life and playing it safe. You are hiding from negative emotions. This is silly. Negative emotions are nothing to be afraid of. They are simply an aspect of your inner guidance system. You want to know when you are looking at something from a perspective that doesn't serve you. You want to be sensitive to these feelings. You want to be able to identify these signals from inside. You can truly appreciate your guidance system because this is how you alter your perspective and reduce the effects of limiting beliefs.

Imagine changing your approach to life and instead of worrying about conditions where negative emotion might arise, you actually look forward to feeling negative emotion. How would this even be possible? If you truly understood that a negative emotion is just a signal that you have a limiting belief and you could analyze these beliefs, prove them false, and thereby make real change, which then creates a better-feeling reality, then you would want to encounter as much negative emotion as possible. If every time you felt bad you could wipe away the limiting belief that caused you to feel bad, then your life would improve as a result of every encounter with a bad-feeling emotion.

The reality is that everything you truly want is available to you right now; it's just that you have these limiting beliefs that cause resistance and this resistance keeps all of your desires from entering your reality. If you had no limiting beliefs, everything you wanted would come to you instantaneously.

Let us give you an example of how desire and limiting beliefs work. You have the desire to go to a nice restaurant for dinner. You have very little resistance to this desire because you have reduced your limiting beliefs to such an extent that they are hardly resistant at all. Therefore, dinner at a nice restaurant is something you can manifest easily.

What else is fairly easy for you to manifest? Can you manifest a movie?

Change Made on the Inside Creates a New Reality on the Outside

Do you like going to the movies? Is this a desire where there are very few limiting beliefs and thus it is easily manifested? Can you manifest a weekend trip to a nearby city? Do you like taking little road trips and spending a couple of days out of town? This can be manifested easily if you have few limiting beliefs. Can you manifest a vacation in Italy for a month? There might be a few limiting beliefs around this and so this desire may take a bit of planning and preparation before it manifests. Could you manifest a less expensive trip to Italy and make it a week rather than a month? This might be more plausible given your set of limiting beliefs.

Your life is created by how you feel on the inside. Your limiting beliefs are a true representation of your fears. These fears are irrational and are therefore false. However, unless you analyze them and prove they are false, they remain true for you. Your life will remain limited. You will not be able to manifest what you desire because your limiting beliefs cause resistance. Realize that negative emotion is simply a gift from the universe that will help you identify limiting beliefs as they arise. The rest is up to you. This is how you make real change. Your reality changes to reflect the real change you've made by doing the work necessary to reduce the intensity of limiting beliefs.

Limiting beliefs will always exist. Once you've adopted one, it's with you forever. The strength of the limiting belief will cause you to resist your desire, but if your desire is stronger than your limiting beliefs, you will overcome obstacles in the path to the manifestation of your desire.

You have some limiting beliefs about going out to a nice restaurant for dinner, but they are weak and so there is little resistance within them. This desire is easily and often manifested. All you have to do is reduce the intensity of all limiting beliefs and everything you want will manifest in the most elegant way possible. You can also increase the strength of your desire so that the obstacles in your path will not seem so big.

Very strong desire will overcome strong and entrenched limiting beliefs. If you have ever heard a story of a mother who lifted a car off her child, this is an example of a very strong desire overcoming very strong limiting beliefs. Any desire will be manifested by the universe as long as it is stronger than the limiting beliefs. You can have, be, and do anything you want in this reality as long as your desire is more robust than your limiting beliefs. Increase the power of your desires while simultaneously reducing the intensity of your limiting beliefs.

Your desire is really up to you. The universe will help you reduce your limiting beliefs by placing you in situations where you have the opportunity to confront them and, through analysis, reduce their intensity. Reduce the intensity of your limiting beliefs and you automatically increase the chances that your desire will manifest.

Have you ever heard of a story where someone had birthed a desire and then forgot about it? Several months later the desire manifested seemingly out of nowhere and the person was quite surprised. How did this happen? The universe simply presented events designed to reduce the person's limiting beliefs and gradually the intensity of those beliefs were lowered to the point where the desire became stronger than the beliefs and the desire manifested. A very strong desire will manifest as soon as the limiting beliefs are reduced to the point where they can no longer hold the person away from that which they desire. The speed at which this is accomplished is up to the person and their ability to manage their belief system.

You have an advantage. You now understand how this system works. You can engage the art of analysis anytime you encounter negative emotion. You can reduce the intensity of your limiting beliefs and move through the fear. You can increase the intensity of your desire so that you'll have an easier time overcoming obstacles. You have a newfound power to create the reality you prefer.

III.

The first inner change you must make is your approach to negative emotion. If you can see negative emotion as a signal flare alerting you to the presence of a limiting belief, you can literally accomplish anything you want. When you shy away from negative emotion because you can't handle the pain and distress, you play it too safe. By playing it safe out of fear of negative emotion, you actually diminish the intensity and strength of your desires.

Let's say you truly desire a mate and this desire is very strong. You look in the mirror and you pick apart what you see with judgment and scrutiny that is based on years of feeling unworthy. You believe that you are not attractive enough to find a mate who will love you. When these thoughts occur to you, you feel negative emotion. So what are you really doing? You are reducing the intensity of your desire and you are increasing the intensity of your limiting beliefs. You are creating what you do not want by focusing on conditions in the moment that you do not like. Your future reality is being created from this very low-vibrational place.

From this place, you decide to do something to change the conditions in the attempt to manifest a mate. Remember, if you change the conditions on the outside without changing the conditions on the inside, the outer change will not last. Also, the change will be painful and difficult. The results will be paltry by comparison and your feelings will not substantially improve.

Let's say you go on a calorie-restricted diet and you lose twenty pounds. You take another look in the mirror and you see the improvement and this causes you to feel good. You are looking at yourself in a way that aligns with how your inner self sees you and as a result you feel positive emotion. You put on some new clothes and you go out with friends. You meet someone and start up a conversation. Your desire to find a mate has caused you to make a change to the outer conditions and as a result, you have a little more confidence. You meet a new person and start dating.

Suddenly, the new person does something and your immediate reaction is to take offense. Maybe they don't return your calls or texts quickly enough and you choose a perspective that is based on the same limiting belief, i.e. that you are not attractive enough. You feel negative emotion, which is the indication that this belief is still present and you sink into a low-emotional state of being. You might now receive an urge to do something in order to ease the pain of how you are feeling. But the action you take will be contrary to what you really want and so you do something that puts an end to this budding romance. You just created a reality you did not want.

Because you had not made the change on the inside, but rather believed that all you needed to do was make a change to the outer conditions, your change could not and did not last. You might have kept it going for a few weeks, months, or even years, yet eventually everything would unravel because the inner change was never made. Change the inside, not the outside. Change who you are being and move toward who you really are.

We will concede that from your perspective it seems much easier to change the outer conditions than it is to change how you approach life. You have always striven to make changes to the conditions in your life. You have done everything in order to create nice conditions and to constantly improve them. You believe that this is an effective approach to life.

We understand that this is how it appears; however, it just doesn't make sense given what we know of the laws of the universe.

You believe that in order to feel good, everything and everyone must appeal to your positive judgment. You want a nice place to live, so you buy a house, fix it up, furnish it, and make it as nice as you can. When something breaks, you stop feeling good and you react to the problem by feeling negative emotion. So you fix the thing that breaks and you return to feeling good.

When you find a mate that you love, you feel good. However, when your mate does something you do not like, you react by being angry or upset and you tell your mate not to do that again. You seek to change the behavior of other people so you can feel good. If your mate changes the behavior, you return to feeling good. If not, you feel bad all over again. You allow your mate's behavior to control how you feel.

When you go to work, you behave in a manner that produces positive responses from your boss. If you do something she dislikes and she says something to you about it, you react by feeling bad. You alter your behavior so that she keeps praising you until something happens and her praise is suspended. If you cannot maintain a level of behavior that keeps the praise coming, you might eventually quit your job. You can't control your boss, so you can't be sure that negative emotion won't keep coming and the only way to solve this problem is by finding a new job.

When you live a life dictated by your positive and negative reaction to the outside conditions of your life, you are leaving how you feel in the hands of others. If the conditions are good, you choose to feel good, but if they are bad, you will always choose to feel bad. Mostly you feel good, so you tend to accept the times when you do not feel good and you believe that this is just how life is. It could be worse.

We are here to explain to you that the universe is a system and that system was designed for you to expand your conscious awareness through joyful experience. Can every experience, even those contrasting ones, be joyful? Absolutely. You can live a life leveraging the powers of the universe to create a joyful life and still expand every step of the way. Expansion does not have to be painful. How you react to unpleasant situations is the only thing that causes you pain. How you perceive the conditions is what brings up negative emotion. How you view negative emotion is the only reason you fear it. Learn to understand that negative emotion is not a bad thing, it is simply a message. When you understand this concept, the pain associated with negative emotion dissipates.

IV.

Imagine if you could never feel negative emotion. What would life be like? It would be like driving a car without a steering wheel. You would not get very far. Without your guidance system, you would not be able to create your reality and you would not be able to expand your consciousness. These are two fundamental aspects of physical reality. This is why you came. You came to expand your consciousness and to create your own reality. Without emotions, you could not do either.

You might think it would be preferable never to feel hatred ever again and we might agree with you. The feeling of hatred is a very intense negative emotion and it carries with it a lot of pain. It is highly unpleasant because it indicates the presence of a very intense limiting belief. The belief says that unless the subject of my hatred is removed from my life, I can never feel good again. Even if it is removed, I will still have a hard time feeling good. So you will do whatever it takes to remove the object of your hatred from the conditions that surround you. We ask you this: when you feel hatred, are you inspired to change the outer conditions or the inner conditions?

There are few people on Earth who would first seek to change how they are feeling before they try to change the outside conditions. The vast majority of people living today would rather change the thing that brings up hatred (or any other emotion) than the perspective that causes them to hate something. You see, it is all a mental exercise and it has nothing to do with the thing; it always has to do with you.

There is a group of people known as terrorists who would gladly sacrifice their lives just to inflict a little pain on the subject of their hatred. From their perspective, Western culture has caused them to suffer and they want retribution. It feels to them that the only way for them to feel better is to seek vengeance. Their emotional state of being is so low that they only have access to these-low vibrational thoughts and ideas. Their fear is so great that they cannot allow themselves to choose another more empowering perspective. They are ignoring their guidance system and deliberately creating the lives they do not want.

When you choose a perspective that will create a reality you do not want, you will be alerted by your inner self and you will feel negative emotion. The more limiting the perspective, the stronger the emotion. If you really feel bad, it's because you are looking at something from a seriously limiting perspective and your inner self is sending you a very strong warning urging you to find a more empowering perspective. You are in the act of creating your reality when you choose a perspective that has the potential to attract what you do not want. If you maintain this perspective, you will be inspired to action that is completely out of alignment with who you really are and the life you really want. Either change your perspective or suffer the consequences.

Have you ever been angry and said or did something you later regretted? Those words and actions had a significant impact on your life. If you had not said them, your life might have unfolded differently. In the heat of the moment, you chose a perspective that was out of alignment with what you really wanted and you said something that changed the course of your life forever. Once the words are said or the action is taken, your life changes as a result. In moments of anger, you often say and do things that are in conflict with the life you really want. If you could see what was happening in the moment from a more empowering, higher, and broader perspective, you would not feel so bad and you would not succumb to low-vibrational urges.

If you can understand the essence of what we are talking about here, you can change your prejudice against negative emotion. Negative emotion is simply a warning. It is not a bad thing. You do not have to live safely in the hope that you will avoid facing negative emotion. Learn to accept it for what it is. Learn to feel it and immediately analyze it. Learn to adjust your perspective on the spot. The reason you want to avoid negative emotion is because you allow it to linger and you brood and sulk over it. Once you learn to deal with every negative emotion in the instant it pops up, you won't feel nearly as bad for nearly as long. The fear of the negative emotion will be dissipated.

V.

How you react to something sets forth a new path toward a new future. Reaction is a choice. This choice will determine which path you take. When you react negatively, depending on the power of your thoughts, words, and actions, you will go down a path toward what you do not want. When you react negatively, you begin to create negatively. Change your reaction to how you perceive things and you will regain control of your most important creation: your life.

Currently, something happens and you unconsciously choose a perspective and that perspective causes you to feel good, bad, or somewhere in between. It is a habit of reaction. You aren't thinking; you're just reacting. You are not analyzing the situation; you are simply allowing your prejudice and judgment to cloud your perception. When you perceive something to be bad or wrong and you react negatively, you are choosing a reaction based in fear. How you react to something then leads to the next moment and the next moment. Your reactions build momentum and it is from this place that you create your future.

A reaction is a very powerful statement. It is a declaration. This is good and that is bad. How you react to something causes a shift in your consciousness. Your reaction creates the reception of certain specific channels of thought. It's like tuning into a radio station. There are many, many channels to choose from. Negative reactions give you access to many varieties of fear-based channels. Positive reactions give you access to the love-based channels.

If you have a negative reaction, you are choosing to tune yourself to one of the channels that is based in fear. This means that the thoughts and ideas that are mostly available to you in the moment resonate with the fear you are feeling. The thoughts you think, the words you are inclined to speak, and most of the actions available to you are based in fear. They are designed to relieve the negative feelings associated with the reaction. So, when you react negatively in the moment to anything, you are most likely to think a thought about changing the outside condition.

It could be something very mild. You could be bored and decide to go and watch TV or open the fridge. You are trying to change the outer condition by finding something outside of you that will change how you feel. You feel uncomfortable in your boredom, so you seek anything that will quickly and easily relieve the feeling. You reach for a piece of cake and you change your state. However, the piece of cake is not aligned with what you truly want or who you really are. It does nothing to move you toward the life you desire; rather, it takes you in the opposite direction.

You will look at this example and tell yourself that it's no big deal. So what if you have a piece of cake or watch TV? It's just one insignificant piece and it doesn't really have any impact. We agree, but this is a habit of behavior that involves momentum and it is detrimental. The approach to life where one seeks outside distractions in order to soothe inside feelings leads to a limited and less desirable life experience.

Now, let's say that this approach to life worked for you. Let's imagine that if you were to feel bored and you looked for an outside condition to change your low-emotional state of being, you decided to do twenty push-ups. We would agree that this response to your inner feeling would be a positive response and would be in line with what you truly want. However, the positive thought is not as available to you as the negative thought unless you are able to stop and think about it. Reactions are quick and are created in the moment. They are habitual. You tend to react consistently positive or negative depending on the situation. In the moment of a negative reaction, you will likely go with the first thought, which will be one that matches your reaction. It will be negative.

Now let's imagine that you absolutely understood the concept that a negative reaction created the pathway to a channel of fear-based thoughts and ideas. You further understood that when you entertain these fear-based thoughts, you create a future reality that is also fear-based. When you choose to speak words or take action based in fear, you are creating a life that you do not want. You are moving away from being who you really are.

There is a way to consciously and creatively deal with this issue. First, you can choose how you react to anything. The instant you feel negative emotion, you can stop and think. Why am I feeling this way? Why do I think it is wrong? How does it help me to see that it is wrong? Could I find a more empowering perspective? Could I see this in a way that aligns with what I really want and who I really am? Can I give up my fear? Can I understand that this is happening for me, not to me? Can I change the way I feel rather than trying to change the other person or the outside conditions? Now that I have chosen to look at it in a way that serves me, do I feel relief?

If you knew that nothing ever happens to you, but that it always happens for you, you could learn to analyze every condition. With this perspective in mind, you would regain access to love-based channels and you could make decisions based in love. You would have access to empowering thoughts and your actions would be inspired from a place of feeling good. You would stop sabotaging yourself and you would engage the leverage of universal powers. You would be unstoppable.

There are two spectrums of thought available to you at any moment in time. If you feel good, you have access to a wide range of love-based thoughts and ideas depending on how good you feel. When you are fully engaged in your passion, be it art, music, business, conversation, research, etc., you have access to the very top of the spectrum. In these times of bliss, you are a vibrational match to high-vibrational thoughts and ideas. However, when you are feeling bad, when you are sad, angry, depressed, bored, or upset, you have access to the lower end of the spectrum. The thoughts available to you are generally based in fear. When you receive inspiration (in the form of an urge), it will be to do something to make yourself feel better, but because you have access to low-vibrational thoughts that resonate with how you feel, you will do and say things that do not engage universal forces and will be counter to everything you want in life.

When you learn to react with curiosity rather than judgment, you poke holes in the lower channels. When you seek to analyze your thoughts, understanding that they come from the lower channels, you can prevent yourself from acting in ways that are detrimental. Instead, you can reach for higher-vibrational thoughts and a more empowering perspective. You can slowly pull yourself out of victimhood and back into your original state of the conscious creator.

It all starts by changing the way you react to everything outside of you. Don't try to change the outer conditions; go inside and change your own channel. Stop and analyze your thoughts. Are they leading you to action that aligns with love or fear? If the actions are based in fear, you will create what you do not want. If the actions are based in love, you are consciously creating the life you prefer.

VI.

If you found yourself in a state of fear and you could stop and analyze the situation and see that the fear is false because it is irrational, then you could choose a higher perspective and reach for love-based thoughts. These thoughts would then lead you to other love-based thoughts, words, and inspired action. When you do not analyze your fear at the base of any negative emotional state, you allow in fear-based thoughts that resonate with how you are feeling in the moment. These thoughts lead to other fear-based thoughts, words, and uninspired actions such as urges and compulsions, which create the life experience you do not desire.

When you feel lonely, it is because there is an irrational fear that is the basis of that feeling. The feeling of loneliness could not arise within you unless there was fear. This fear is irrational because you cannot die from loneliness. The loneliness that you are experiencing is not life-threatening. It is an irrational fear and therefore it is false. You are feeling a fear and taking a perspective that is out of alignment with the truth, with who you really are, and with the laws of the universe.

Let's examine the irrational fear of loneliness. You compare yourself to others and you feel lonely. You believe that you require physical people to be around you more than they are. You believe that something must be wrong with you, otherwise you would not be lonely. You might even believe that it is the fault of some condition outside yourself. However, there is nothing to fear, there is nothing wrong with you, there is nothing wrong with anyone else, and the fear is simply false. The feeling of loneliness is simply a perspective you decide to adopt. Now, how do you react to this feeling?

If you are an unconscious creator, you allow the perspective and the bad feeling to linger. You don't know any better. You seek relief from the feeling, but you don't understand it because you haven't analyzed it. You let the feeling build and it gains momentum over time. All you have access to are thoughts and ideas that resonate with loneliness. The thoughts revolve around why you are lonely, what's wrong with you, and what's wrong with everyone else. You want to feel better so you attempt to alter your state of being by reaching for something outside of you. You will either reach for some stimulant like food, drink, drug, smoke, etc. or you might take a nap. The nap would be the only choice here that would be in line with what you truly wanted.

Now, let's examine the feeling of loneliness from the perspective of the conscious creator. You feel lonely and you notice the negative emotion because you are so used to feeling good that this feels really off. You stop in the moment and you become curious. Why do I have these feelings? What is the purpose of this emotion? Where has my perspective taken me? What is the fear at the basis of this limiting belief? The fear is that I should have more people around me, I should be more sociable, I should be more lovable. I should be different than I am so that others will love me. This fear is irrational and it is false.

I can prove it's false by providing mountains of evidence that tell me I am sociable, I am lovable, and I do not need to be anything other than who I am. I have friends, I work with people, and I have some people in my life who do love me. I love others and that is what is most important. I will attract more friends and love more people when needed, but for now I am happy with the friends I have.

The fear-based perspective leads to low-vibrational thoughts that seek to change outside conditions first. The love-based perspective is aligned with thoughts that seek to change the feeling first. When the feeling is elevated and a higher channel is accessed, you will receive inspired thoughts, words, and actions. In the lower channels, you received thoughts about eating food to relieve your state of being. In the higher channels, you receive an inspired thought to phone an old friend. The lower channels provide you with thoughts that tend to lead you away from what is wanted and the higher channels tend to provide you with inspired thought that leads you toward what is wanted.

Notice here that the inspired thought does lead to a change in the conditions. You receive the thought to call your friend and this phone call makes you feel better. But you choose to feel better first and then take action that was inspired from a place of feeling better. When you do not do the work to feel better first, you take action from a bad-feeling place and the result will be the attraction of outside conditions that match how you feel. It is simply the Law of Attraction at work.

The reason you cannot lose the weight you want to lose is because you do not choose to elevate your emotional state of being before you take action. You just react to the emotion and take action that is inspired from a low-vibrational state of being. This action is a low-vibrational action and tends to be counter-productive. You cannot receive what you want when you consistently sabotage your desires by acting from fear-based positions. You must improve your state of being before taking action.

It doesn't matter what your issue is. It could be money, relationships, health, work, love, weight, addiction, etc. If you continue to take action from a low emotional state, you will continue to do and say things that move you away from what you truly want. You might make great progress toward your dreams and desires, then suddenly something happens that gives rise to irrational fear and you say or do something that ceases your forward momentum and brings you back where you started.

Imagine being an alcoholic. You resist the temptation to drink for many days in a row and you are feeling good. Then something happens to cause

103

fear and you are inspired to take action to relieve the negative emotion. From your low-emotional state, the action you are inspired to do is to have a drink. If you can see what is happening in the moment and reach for another, better-feeling perspective and analyze the fear for what it is, you will elevate your state of being. Once you've gotten hold of a more empowering perspective, you will receive thoughts that align with that. Now, instead of taking a drink to soothe your feelings, you receive the thought to go to a meeting or call your sponsor. This is an example of the different channels of thought available from different emotional states of being.

Changing your state of being is an inner change. Change made from the inside affects the outside conditions. You have the knowledge and the tools you need to make significant inner changes that then utilize the forces of the universe to create the life experience you truly desire. It is all a matter of perspective and this is an approach to life that is in full alignment of universal laws.

When you attempt to change the conditions around you without changing your own vibration, the change will always be temporary. Lasting change is made by first altering the way you feel. When you feel good, you receive thoughts that resonate with how you feel and you say words and take action that is inspired by these good-feeling thoughts. The words you say and the actions you take will change the conditions around you and the changes will last. If you want a lean body, learn to feel good about the body you have now, about the life you have now, and about the conditions that exist now. If you can't feel good in this moment in time, then you will have difficulty feeling good in the future.

Chapter Nine

How Your Thoughts Affect Your Weight (and Everything Else)

In this reality, nothing is more powerful than thought. The thoughts you think create the life you live. It's as simple as this. It is the fundamental design of the system of physical reality. You are here to practice your powers of creation by choosing thoughts that align with what you want. Every thought you think is a point of creation. Every thought affects what you are creating. Every thought has the power to add to the momentum or to slow it down. You attract thoughts and then you think them. You have total control over the thoughts you think even though you might believe otherwise.

If you were to describe where your thoughts come from, you might tell us that they are created in your mind. This is not true. Your mind is not a thought factory. If it were, would you create all these random, swirling thoughts that fill your head in every single moment of every day? If you constructed thoughts in your mind, wouldn't they be more defined? Wouldn't there be some sort of structure? Think about a factory that makes cars. Raw materials go in one end, people or robots put them together in an organized fashion, and the finished car emerges out the other end.

If your mind was a thought factory, the raw materials of thought would come in from somewhere and then your mind would assemble that into coherent and structured thought. Basically, every thought would be like every other thought. This would not work in this reality. In order to create, you must have access to every possible thought. You must be able to access new thoughts.

Think of your mind as a shortwave radio that can receive and transmit signals. Like a radio, your mind is tuned to wavelengths or vibrations, or channels of thought. Depending on your vibrational level, you have access to various channels. Some channels are accessed at low vibrations and others are accessed at very high vibrational frequencies. We, as Joshua, broadcast from a very high vibrational frequency. In order to find us and understand what we are saying, you must be tuned to our channel.

Once you hear what we have to say, you can then recall it and think about it any time you like as long as you are still in that frequency range. When you dip down to a lower vibration, you will find it is not as easy to hear or understand our message. As soon as you regain your high vibration, you are able to hear us once again. It works like this with all thought.

All the thoughts and ideas that have ever been thought still exist. All the thoughts and ideas that ever will be thought also exist. Thoughts that have not yet been thought are at frequencies that have not yet been reached. They may be reached tomorrow or never, but they still exist. When you get an original idea, it's not that you created the idea, it's just that you were the first to reach the vibrational frequency of the idea. Once you've unlocked the idea and you send it out to the world in the form of an invention or a book, then others may resonate with that idea because they too have reached that vibrational level.

Gary reached a vibrational level with us and from this we created Joshua. Joshua is the combination of our teachings and Gary's translation. If he had not reached vibrational alignment with us, Joshua would not exist. If another were to reach vibrational alignment with us (and many have) and if they were able to translate our message through the filter of their perspective, it would be called something else.

You have reached a vibrational level high enough to hear Joshua's message and to incorporate the teachings into your life. Something caused you to reach for this high vibration. In this case, it might have been your desire to create a lean body. The desire led you to a series of steps that resulted in the discovery of this book. If you were not a vibrational match to this book, you would not be reading it now.

However, it is also likely that your desire to create a healthy and lean body was just one of the steps necessary to raise your vibration enough to find this material. You might have been in the vibrational frequency range of our teachings, which have been available for some time now. Yet, until this book was written on this particular subject, you did not allow yourself to find us before. Our message is available in many places, but your resistance was not eased enough until you read the title of this book. While you might truly want to create a lean body, and this is the reason you bought the book, what you really want to do is create a wonderful life experience that encapsulates every area of your life.

II.

If you could control the quality of every single thought that comes to you, what would that really mean? It would mean that you were a deliberate creator of your life. Since your thoughts create your reality, if you could maintain a vibration where you received only high-vibrational thoughts, your life would be created in a way that perfectly aligned with the quality of thoughts you were thinking. You would enjoy a high-quality life experience.

Conversely, If you had absolutely no control over the thoughts you think, then what could you do to create a better life? You would have to control your emotional state of being so that you could access good-quality thoughts by feeling good. If this were possible (which it is), you would also be able to create a high-quality life experience. But unfortunately it is not really possible to control every thought you think or every emotion you feel. This is a good thing. You wanted to come here to sift through it all to discover what it is you like and what you do not like. You are here to joyfully explore certain aspects of physical reality. You are on a journey of discovery. It is really a journey of self-discovery.

If you could control every thought, you could create a high-quality life and if you could control your state of being in every moment, you could also create a high-quality life. But you don't need to control every thought and every feeling in every moment. This would be exhausting. You would be trapped in this prison of thought control. You could not explore. You would be too focused on controlling your thoughts. You do not need to control your thoughts because you have a guidance system. Whenever you think a low-quality thought, your guidance system kicks in and sends you a signal in the form of negative emotion. You don't have to pay attention to your thoughts because your guidance system is constantly aware of every thought you are thinking and if you choose a thought that does not align with what you want, you will be notified.

Isn't this an excellent system? You can think any thought you like and if you choose a thought that doesn't help you in your journey toward your desire, your guidance system lets you know it. This means you are completely free to take any position or adopt any perspective. You just choose the one that seems to fit and if it doesn't fit, you will receive a little nudge and then you can choose a new perspective.

If you had no desires, you could think any thought and it would not matter. You would receive no emotion. It would not matter what you believe, what you think, or how you feel. If you had zero desire, there would be no need for guidance. Guidance exists only to keep you on track. Your emotions let you know if you are moving toward your desires or away from them. You can choose any desire you like. You could choose to help others or blow up buildings, it does not matter to the universe. If you have a desire, you will be guided there through your emotions.

When you think a thought that does not feel good, what do you think that means? It means that the thought you are entertaining in this moment is not one that will move you toward your desire. It is a fear-based thought. It means that maybe you are afraid of reaching your desire. What will it look like once you've realized your dream? Will it be worth it? Will you like it? Is it too far away? Should you give up and try for something smaller? Thoughts that resonate with fear feel bad because they take you further away from your desire.

Is this a bad thing? Not at all. But it is based in fear and if the dream does not have the potential to kill you or injure your body, then the fear is irrational. If it's an irrational fear, then it's false. However, you may be asking a deeper question. What if you achieve your dream and it's not to your liking? What if it's not good? What will you do then? What if you make the wrong choice?

Your choices don't cause your dream to happen. You don't make a series of choices that lead to the manifestation of your desire. It's not that black and white. You see, from your limited perspective, it is not really possible to map a route to your desire. The universe creates many, many routes and in each turn you either move toward it or away from it. But your choices don't really have that much of an impact.

When you look back on anything you've accomplished in your life, you see a specific route that you took. You look at pivotal moments in your life and you think that certain specific decisions brought you to the manifestation of your desire. If it seemed like a good decision, then you call it right. If it seemed like a bad decision then you call it wrong. They are not good or bad, right or wrong; they were just the steps. If you had made different decisions in those specific moments, it would not have mattered. You would have come to the same place.

Your vibration creates the route, not your decisions. You are faced with countless decisions every day. There are so many decisions that if you make a wrong one now, there are many right ones that you can make in the future. If you miss one step now, you will be presented with many opportunities later. There is no luck. You get where you get because your vibration creates a million paths to it.

So if there are millions of choices and therefore millions of routes, how do you really contribute to the eventual manifestation of a desire? If you are drawn by your vibration along a twisty and windy path that will inevitably lead to your desire, what can you do to aid the process and make the journey a little less bumpy? You can pay attention to your guidance system and allow yourself to make adjustments to your thoughts, beliefs, and perspective every step of the way.

Let's imagine that you have a desire to find a mate and create a family. Once you have birthed this desire, the universe goes to work. You are like a piece of clay that must be molded. You are a single person with a set of beneficial and limiting beliefs. You have a certain approach to life. You have a certain set of unique qualities, attributes, and features. You may have a very specific desire. You may have been thinking about this most of your life. So how will the universe mold you into a person who is ready for their desire to manifest? The universe will have to go to work on you. You will be transformed.

The single version of you is very different from the married version of you. You have few responsibilities now. Your outlook on life is very different as a single person. You are younger. You are less experienced. You understand less about yourself and the world. You don't really know what you want yet. Try to imagine the transformation as it takes place over several years. See yourself as the young, inexperienced single version and imagine your path from who you were then to who you would become in a few short years. It's like the transformation from caterpillar to butterfly.

This journey could be joyful and fun or painful and difficult. Guess who's choice that is? That's right; you either make this journey fun and easy or you insert friction and make it difficult and painful.

Let's say that in order for you to rendezvous with the person you would ultimately marry, you would first need the experience of four other relationships. These relationships are critical, because without them, you could not evolve into the person who would match the one you will marry. If you don't experience these other relationships first, you won't be ready for your spouse when the time comes. These four relationships are crucial to your path and therefore they are inevitable. They are coming and you can either enjoy them or resist them.

You might look back at your own relationships and realize that had you not experienced them you would not be who you are now. You would be different. You were changed as a result of them. It may have felt painful at the time, but that was just your own resistance. You could have had fun and felt no resistance. Why were you resistant? Fear. Fear causes you to resist the path toward where you want to go.

Imagine your very first relationship. Did you ever get upset with the other person? Were there any fights? How did you feel when the relationship ended? Each time you were upset, you felt fear and you resisted what was happening. When you got into a fight, you wanted the other person to change so that you could feel better. When you broke up, you felt fear that you might not reach your dream of being married and having a family. If there was no fear, you could have enjoyed this relationship for the duration of its existence. You could have had fun. You could have expanded joyfully.

Do you see now that there was no reason for fear? The relationship was simply a stepping stone designed to move you further along a path that led you to your eventual spouse. Now, having said all that, there might have been some benefit to the contrast because it helped you more narrowly define your desire and it also increased the intensity of your desire. But the pain associated with the contrast made some changes of their own to your belief system. You might have become hardened by the experience. You might have created some defenses that didn't necessarily serve you. In the end there is nothing wrong with a little resistance, but it's not necessary because you are being moved toward your desire. All the resistance does is make the trip a little bumpier and less fun.

III.

When you believe that you know how to get from where you are now to the eventual manifestation of your desire, you are attempting to create a reality based on limited information. You think you know how everything should unfold. When things don't turn out as you hoped or expected, you feel negative emotion. You get upset. The reason you are feeling negative emotion is because of fear. When you expect one thing to happen and something else happens instead, you feel fear. You believe that it was wrong to happen this way. However, you really can't imagine how all of this will unfold and so you are simply making it all up.

When you feel irrational fear, the fear is false so you are fabricating a perspective that causes you to feel fear. You could just as easily don a perspective that allows you to feel good. But the fear causes you to adopt the limiting perspective. Since you made it all up anyway, since you cannot know which path the universe is taking you, since you cannot know how it will all unfold, why not substitute fear for faith?

Imagine going on a roller coaster for the first time. You slowly climb the first steep hill and as you do, you feel anxious. What's going to happen when you get to the top of the incline? You're going to descend very quickly. The roller coaster is designed to be scary, but since you rationally understand that it's relatively safe, you have faith that you will survive the ride. Most people survive roller coaster rides and therefore you can adopt the faith that everything will work out just fine and the ride will be fun.

We are here to tell you that your life is like a roller coaster and that is by design. If you knew what was coming, the game would not be any fun. So it's fun not to know what the day will bring. It's fun to explore certain aspects of physical reality. It's fun that things cannot be predicted. When you try to figure out what's going to happen next, well, that's fun too. When you become attached to your predictions, you cause yourself pain when the ride takes an unexpected turn. Release your attachments to your predictions. If things turn out differently than you expected, believe that it's for your highest good.

When you were involved in your first love, there were times when you wanted the other person to be different than they were. If only they could be like this, then things would be good. The first time you were dumped in a relationship, you felt pain. You might have thought at the time, "If only the person loved me, things would have been different." Looking back, would you really have wanted to stay with that person or could you appreciate the growth that that relationship created? You think you know what you want, but you really don't. When you try to create your own life as you see a specific path in your imagination, you are simply resisting the path that the universe has chosen for you.

So let's talk more about that. You have lived so many years on this planet and you have created a set of very specific desires. Can you describe them to us? If you thought about it for a bit, you might speak for a few minutes listing some things you want. You might be quite detailed in your description. But when you compare your verbal description of your desire to the intimate and detailed enormity of your desire that is held within your vibration, it would be like comparing a pamphlet to a library. Your vibration contains it all, from the broad and voluminous idea of your desire to the subtlest nuance. The universe responds to your vibration, not your words. Thank goodness for that!

You must have a set of personal experiences in order to become the version of you that will be ready for your desire. You must undergo a transformation. All of these experiences are for your higher good. They are all part of the transformation process. Most of the experiences will seem good and some will seem bad, but if you can understand that they are all for your higher good and they are all part of the transformation process, then you can begin to judge them all as good rather than seeing some of them as wrong.

If you judge an experience as good when it seems wrong, you are going with the flow of the transformation. You are showing little resistance. You are altering your emotional state of being on your own and you are entering the state of allowing. When you allow these experiences to occur without negative judgment, you move swiftly through them and they cause you little to no pain. Isn't that a helpful perspective?

Imagine reliving your entire first relationship in an emotional state of allowing. Your former boyfriend or girlfriend could do nothing to cause you to be upset. You know that how they are being is just fine because you have no fear. You realize that this first relationship was set up to give you certain experiences you needed in order to become the person who would be ready for your future spouse. If you could not feel fear, you could not feel negative emotion. With no fear, the only thing left would be the fun parts. The only problem with this scenario is that you would be living as the evolved version of yourself and you would be expressing unconditional love. If there is no fear, then there can only be unconditional love. Your former flame would probably behave quite differently in the presence of unconditional love.

The point we are making here is that you can't know where your path will lead you. All you can know is that every experience is for your highest good, even if it seems bad or wrong at the time. From the higher perspective or even after a bit of time, you will be able to see that the experience was good and right all along. It may have seemed bad in the moment, but it really wasn't. Release your fear of the conditions and of these experiences and realize that you are simply being transformed because you have a desire and you are willing to take the journey. It's just a journey and it's supposed to be fun.

IV.

Did you know that your thoughts control your weight and nothing else? Did you know that you created a perception of who you are and that your thoughts always align with your perception? Did you know you could alter your perception of yourself if you wanted to? It's true. You have created a perception of who you are. Through all your experiences, you've developed a persona. This persona is not real; it's completely imaginary. No one else sees you like you see yourself.

Your fabricated persona is comprised of certain specific personality traits, physical features, and mental constructs. The one thing to always keep in mind is that your persona is not true. Who you think you are is not who you really are. Your persona is a smaller and limited version of who you really are. In actuality, it's minuscule compared to the magnificence that is you. This is true of everyone.

No one lives in physical reality as the fullest expression of who they really are, however, everyone is on a path toward the highest version of themselves. Right now, in this moment, no matter what your life is like or how you feel about yourself, your present state is the most evolved and highest version of you that has ever existed. Yet there is still a long way to go.

If you were to describe yourself, you might say things like "I'm attractive, I'm young, I'm intelligent, I'm tall, I'm funny, I'm articulate, and I'm a people person." You might go on to say, "Sometimes I'm impatient, irritable, moody, unfocused, and irresponsible." However you describe yourself, it is your unique description and that is your persona. If your mother were to describe you, it would be a different description. You father, siblings, mate, children, friends, co-workers, bosses, employees, customers, etc., all have a different idea about who you are. It all depends on the perspective.

Since your persona is fabricated, there's no need to defend it. If you believe yourself to be intelligent and someone challenges you on that, you feel fear because you are concerned that you might not be who you say you are. So when this fear arises in the form of negative emotion, what do you do? You defend yourself and attack the other person and their intelligence. If you had no fear about that aspect of yourself, you could not feel negative emotion and you would have no need to do anything.

Every point of your persona must be defended at all times. If you believe anything good about yourself and that belief is challenged, you will feel fear in the form of negative emotion. This emotion is letting you know that the fear exists, but that fear is false. Stop entertaining thoughts that go against how you perceive yourself. Allow yourself to create a perception that is empowering and when the perception is challenged, realize that the fear is false.

It is good and right to think very highly of yourself because you are the most evolved version of you that has ever existed. You are not better than anyone else, but you are equally as worthy as any other. If you are as worthy as any who ever lived, you may accept that you have some very fine qualities that make you unique to all the world. Go ahead and create as many positive definitions of yourself as you can think of and don't let anyone talk you out of them. You can create any persona, and since all personas are fabricated anyway, why not construct one that perfectly suits who you want to be?

When you recognize your weaknesses, this is not really constructive. The only weakness you have is believing you have a weakness. In reality, you are fully capable of doing anything you truly desire. Now, before we go any further, let's clarify that statement. You might be thinking, "If I'm capable of creating any persona I truly want, then I want to be a pop sensation. Is this possible? Can I go on a talent show being completely tone deaf and become the next superstar?" Our answer is yes and no.

We say that you can have anything you truly desire. If your passion is singing and you love performing in front of an audience, then certainly you can enjoy a life singing to people. Will you be the next big thing? That is all up to you and what you truly want. Being a pop superstar is quite different from being someone who loves singing in front of an audience.

Now, if your desire is to escape your life of poverty and insecurity and what you crave is love and adoration, then you are looking at what is wrong with your life and seeking a way out. This approach is backwards and will not work. Even if you became famous, you would not feel loved and adored. Your focus is on a false desire.

When you believe that you fall short in certain areas, it is simply a limiting belief. If you think you're unattractive, overweight, too tall, too short, or whatever, you are adopting a limited perception of who you are. Think about it. You chose your specific body because this body would help you seek out certain aspects of reality that you intended to explore. Your body is perfect for the life you chose. It is perfect for you. It's your thoughts about it that are simply not aligned with what you truly want. You've adopted some limiting beliefs about yourself and you've incorporated them into your persona.

Let's imagine that your body is perfect for the life you chose to live. Your heritage, your skin color, your hair, eyes, nose, and teeth are all perfect. Your height is perfect as well. When you compare yourself to others, you might judge yourself to be something less in certain areas and you believe that by changing the way you look, you'll change the way you feel. No matter how much you are able to change the look of your body, if you continue your habit of comparison with others, you will always find examples of others who look better than you. Give up the comparison and realize that your body is perfect for your life and it is not interchangeable. Without your exact body, you could not live the life you intended prior to your birth into this environment.

Accept your body as it is. Love your body in its present shape. Be comfortable in your body now and then seek to create an improved physical condition. Move toward what you desire and not away from what you dislike. When you understand that your body was created for you alone, you can modify the shape and condition of it through appreciation and acceptance.

V.

When you feel good, you have access to thoughts that resonate with how you feel. You have access to ideas that align with what you want. If you can focus on how you want your body to feel and you continue to maintain a strong desire to feel good, then you will attract thoughts that will move you toward how you want to feel.

In the past, you have wanted to lose weight because you did not like the way you looked. You compared yourself to others and you felt like your body was not as attractive. You believed that if you lost some weight, you would look better and as a result, you would feel better. But because your desire was more about getting rid of what you did not want (a fat body), you actually attracted thoughts that made losing weight very difficult. This is why you and countless others cannot lose weight easily or keep it off. You are fighting against the most fundamental principle of the universe.

If you can place the focus of your desire on feeling good in your body rather than trying to change how it looks, then you will receive inspiration that will help you create a good-feeling body. When your body feels good, not only will you return to your natural weight and shape, but every cell in your body will be receiving well-being and functioning optimally. You will not only feel good, you will be healthier too. When you feel good and maintain your health, your body will take its natural shape.

Let's say you've decided to focus on how you feel in your body and nothing more. You are not going to weigh yourself or judge any aspect of your physical appearance as bad. You are not going to compare yourself to others. You are going to write lists of appreciation about your body and everything else in your life. You are simply going to focus everything on feeling good. You are going to intend to feel good. Everything you do is going to bring you to your desire of feeling good in your body.

If your intention is to feel good, then you will receive thoughts that align with that. Before reading this book, you wanted to lose weight. You thought a lot about your weight. You may have weighed yourself often, taken your measurements, or noticed how tight your clothes were. Now you are going to think differently about all this.

You are focused on how you feel. Are you now going to wear tight clothes or comfortable clothes? Before you were focused on how you looked rather than how you felt. Are you now going to care about looking good or feeling good? Before you cared about how much you weighed.

Are you now going to care about your weight or how you feel? Trust us, as long as you seek to feel good, everything else will fall into place.

If you care about how you feel and your desire is to feel good, you will be guided to foods that match how you want to feel. You will be inspired to choose restaurants and order meals that will make you feel good. You will be interested in new foods. You might read articles, overhear conversations, or receive new thoughts and ideas, all of which will lead you toward your desire. You might receive inspiration to go for a walk after dinner, or to ride a bike, or to take a yoga class, or to play tennis.

When you seek to lose weight, you are focused on weight and you will receive thoughts, ideas, inspiration, and urges to maintain or increase your weight. Your thoughts revolve around your weight, not how you feel. You might eat really healthy all day, then you receive this overwhelming urge for some ice cream. Your focus has been on weight and since you have not taken in enough food to maintain your weight, you will attract an undeniable urge to eat. You will fool yourself into thinking that it doesn't matter because you've eaten so healthy all day. You do not need more food; you crave more food. The need is not there, but the craving is unrelenting. It's simply that you have not understood what this was before. The urge was given to you so that you could maintain the weight that is the focus of your attention.

The urge is an inspiration to take action in order to create what you have focused your attention on.

The universe does not know what you think is good or bad; it only knows what you are placing your attention on. Your focus is like a spotlight. You can shine it on anything. You can shine it on the things you like or do not like. When you light up subjects you don't like with your focus of attention, the universe assumes you are looking at things you like. Why else would you place a spotlight on something? You must want more of it, otherwise why would you spend so much energy looking at it? So the universe obliges and brings you more of that. How does this all work? The universe will send you thoughts, ideas, inspiration, cravings, and urges, all to help you move toward the object of your attention.

Instead of placing your attention on how you think you look or what you deem to be an inappropriate weight, place your attention on what you want. You could focus your attention on a lean body, but since you do not consider your body to be lean, you will always return to thinking your body is fat and that is where your focus will return every time. Rather than focusing on the desire to become thin, think about how good it feels in your body. Start to appreciate the times when you feel good. Focus all of your attention on how you feel. Make a deliberate choice to feel good. Do things that make you feel good. Notice when your body does not feel good. Realize that the feeling of hunger is not really a bad feeling. In fact, the feeling of hunger can be seen as a good feeling compared to how you feel when you've eaten too much or when you've eaten something that makes you feel bad.

When you feel a little hunger, let it linger a bit. Play with that feeling. Try to see it as a positive message. Try to perceive it as a good sign. When you feel just a little hungry, your senses are alive. Your mind is clear. You will receive thoughts that align with how you feel. Now is the time to eat just enough to relieve the hunger. Do not delay. Look at the new thoughts and ideas that are streaming to you now. Think about how you want to feel before you put anything in your body. Intend to feel good before making a choice. Don't think about how anything will taste; think about how you will feel after eating it. When you choose to feel good, you will make decisions based on whether you think the result will cause you to feel better or worse.

When you think about weight and you make a decision, you are placing your focus on weight. When you choose something to eat, whatever it is will always add to your weight. It doesn't matter if it's a cookie or a salad. This choice has no difference. The result is ultimately the same thing. However, if you think about how you will feel as a result of eating a salad or a cookie, you know which one will make you feel better. The salad and the cookie are similar in calories, yet one will be much more likely to make you feel better as a result of eating it.

If your focus is on weight, you can justify to yourself that the cookie is not much different than the salad. But when you are focused on feeling good, the salad is the only possible choice. It is the choice that will make you feel good. Focus on feeling good and all your decisions will help you continue to feel good. Remove your attention from what is wrong or bad, and you will be inspired to move toward what you really want.

Chapter Ten

Intention Supports Focus

Intention is one of the most powerful tools in the universe. Intention brings your focus onto what is wanted. When you intend for something to happen, the universe understands this within the framework of your vibrational signal. Your focus of attention shines a light on the object of your desire and the universe responds to that. When you intend, you create focus.

You can intend anything you like and as you do, the universe lines up behind you to assist you. You can intend to enjoy the meal in front of you. You can intend to have a wonderful conversation with a friend. You can intend to get along with your family. You can intend to be happy. You can intend to feel good. You can intend to make choices that will benefit you. You can intend to choose a perspective that empowers you.

Have you used the power of intention to create that which you desire? If not, we hope that you will start thinking about how intention works and why it is so important in your quest for any desire. Intention is like a magic wand that has unlimited power to create. When you get good at intending what you want, you will see that there is very little you need to do personally. The universe has the power to work things out for you. When you use the tool of intention, you leverage the powers of the universe.

Intend to feel good. What could be a more powerful intention than that? Everything you think you want is wanted in the hopes that the result will feel good. If you simply intend to feel good, then you will receive experiences that feel good. It doesn't really need to be any more specific than that. The feelings of love, peace, success, security, faith, trust, abundance, freedom, prosperity, relief, ease, and well-being all feel good. If you feel good, then what else is needed?

Most people believe that in order to feel good, something must happen first. Unfortunately, this simply cannot work in an attractive universe. Unless you feel good first, you cannot receive good-feeling experiences. When you focus on what's wrong in your life and you seek to correct that, ultimately, you will receive more of that. You will receive that which you think is wrong as long as you are focusing on what you think is wrong. When you focus on the positive aspects of any situation, no matter how dire, you shine a spotlight on something good and this moves you toward the receiving of what you think is good.

Imagine that you think you would feel good if you just lost a little weight. Since you do not feel good now, you won't feel good as a result of the weight loss. Being overweight is simply one of the things in your life that you blame for feeling bad. It has nothing to do with the weight. You could be happy with this weight. It has to do with something else. It has to do with your habit of thought. Stop looking for reasons to blame the conditions for how you feel and realize that feeling good is something you must intend to do.

I intend to feel good. I intend to do things that support feeling good. I intend to receive inspiration to act when I feel good. I intend to act when I am inspired to, as long as the inspiration comes while I'm feeling good. I intend to reach for better-feeling thoughts. I intend to have faith that good-feeling thoughts will come to me when I feel good. I intend to receive ideas that resonate with feeling good. I intend to do things that keep me feeling good. I intend to make decisions that will cause me to feel good.

When you set your intentions, you align your focus of attention to what is wanted. No one intends to do anything that is not in their best interests; it's just that they do not set the intention in the first place. Setting intentions can become a habit that will help you create the life you truly desire. When you set intentions before you eat, you will be inspired to take actions and make choices that align with those intentions. When you forget to set your intentions, you will be inspired to take actions that are not necessarily in alignment with what you want.

When you look through the lens of a camera, you must bring the subject of your photo into view. You must adjust the focus until it becomes clear and sharp. You must adjust the aperture and check the lighting. It takes a little thought and concentration beforehand, but once you get everything lined up and you take the shot, magical moments are captured in time. The same is true of intentions.

Before you do anything, you can intend for it to go well. Before entering a room, take a few moments to consider what it is you really want and then intend for that to happen. Before you make a phone call, think about what you want and set your intention. Before you speak, intend for your words to clearly convey your message. Before you eat, intend for the food to nourish your body. Before you do anything, think about what it is you want and set your intentions so that the outcome will be aligned with that.

II.

Until now, you may not have considered what it is you really want in every moment. You may have some idea of the things you want, but have you ever thought about why you wanted those things? Would those things make you happy? Would they be fun? Are they important? Are they true to who you really are? If you want to consciously create the life you desire, then you must think more about what it is you want and why you want it.

Why do you want to have a mate, buy a nice house, make lots of money, or lose the weight? You believe that those things are necessary to your happiness. You believe that without these things, you could not be happy. This is a tightly held limiting belief and it's holding you back from the life you truly desire. What if we were to tell you that you will not lose the weight, but you will be happier than you have ever been in your entire life? What if we could see into your future and we knew what was going to happen? If we saw your specific path and we knew beyond a shadow of a doubt that you would create the most wonderful life, a life filled with love, peace, freedom, and joy, but you would never lose the weight, what would you think?

This is an important question to ask yourself. When you create a strong desire and you believe that unless the desire comes, you could never be happy, then you cut yourself off from happiness until the desire is reached. But there is a great flaw in this premise. You cannot be happy then unless you become happy now. Your future is created by your present. If you lose the weight, or find the mate, or win the lottery, or gain the freedom to travel the world, you will not be happy with those things unless you are happy now. Things don't bring happiness. Things may temporarily distract you from what you think is wrong, but eventually, unless you've actually changed, you will revert back to your same old feelings and the things will slip away.

Let's imagine that you are not happy. You want to remove yourself from the feelings of unhappiness and you think, "What shall I do to become happy? I know...I'll find a mate and fall in love." So you seek out a new relationship from the emotional state of unhappiness and you look for someone who can make you happy. Who do you think you'll meet along the way? People who make you feel unhappy. You attract people based on your vibration. If you are vibrating unhappiness, then those who come to you will match you. They will either be unhappy themselves or they will do things that will make you feel even more unhappy. In this environment of physical reality, you get only that which you are a vibrational match to. It is the Law of Attraction.

Could you become happy with yourself if you never lost any weight for the rest of your life? If this is the best your body will ever look, could you be happy with that? Here's the trick; unless you are happy despite the conditions that surround you, you will have tremendous difficulty creating and maintaining the lean and healthy body you desire. When you are so focused on struggling with the body you have and fighting against it every step of the way, your focus is squarely on what you do not like. It is impossible to get to where you want to go while simultaneously focusing on where you do not want to be.

Just let go. Just give in. Just understand that the battle can never be won. The only way to win is through nonresistance. The only way to move forward is by allowing yourself to float gently downstream. You cannot effort and struggle your way to a body that feels good and stays lean. Eventually something will give and all the work will be for nothing. Stop pushing against and start accepting that the only way anything comes to you is when you choose to allow it to come.

Losing weight is like holding up a wall that's about to fall over. You can stand there and prop up the wall for a little while, but eventually you'll become weary and you'll want to do something else. You'll give up and let the wall fall down. You do not have the strength or endurance necessary to keep holding the wall up forever. Sooner or later you'll give up and the wall will come crashing down.

If you had some sort of device that could hold the wall up for you, then you would never again have to think about that wall. The device you choose could hold up the wall indefinitely and do all the work for you. So you find some steel supports and you brace them against the wall. Now the wall is firmly held in place and you can go about doing something that truly interests you. You remove your attention from the wall because the device is holding it in place for you.

The device to lose weight is trust. The mechanism of this device is the power of the universe. Let the universe sculpt your body for you. Intend for the universe to do all the work. You do not need to do anything but remove your attention from the subject of your weight. You do not need to check on the status of your weight. You do not need to focus any attention on the size of your body. You simply intend to feel good and allow the universe to support you by fulfilling that desire.

If you felt good, what would your life look like? If you asked to feel good and the universe responded by bringing you good-feeling experiences, what would some of those experiences be? You would see and do the things that you liked, which would cause you to feel good. You might make new friends. You might have more fun and success at work. You might have more interesting conversations. You might lose a little weight and feel good in your body. If you intended to feel good and then simply allowed good-feeling things to happen to you, then everything would fall into place.

The only sticking point would be when you noticed that certain things you really want haven't shown up yet. When you want something and it has not yet come, you notice its absence and this prevents if from coming because your focus of attention is on the lack of this thing.

You could intend to feel good and watch as so many good-feeling experiences come your way, but if you aren't losing weight, you might notice that and complain about it. Once you do, you go back to holding up that wall. Your attention is focused squarely on the thing you do not want and now you find yourself back in the state of resistance.

We are here to say that if and when you decide to get into the state of happiness and joy, it must not matter that you do not yet have a mate, or a million dollars in the bank, or the freedom to travel, or the body you desire. The only thing that matters is that you feel good. If you can maintain your appreciation of how you feel, then everything else will fall into place. When you notice that so many things are going well, and you truly feel better than ever before but still you haven't lost all the weight you wanted, then you are choosing to go back to that wall and start propping it up all by yourself.

III.

You are not enjoying the game of losing weight because to you it's a struggle and nothing about it is enjoyable. If it's not enjoyable, don't do it. If you are not inspired to join a gym, don't do it. If you are not inspired to go on some fad diet, don't do it. If you are not inspired to start jogging, don't start. Without the inspiration to do something, the action will not work. There is no gain in pain. Anyone who ever said that got something out of the pain. They enjoyed the pain; you don't have to.

When you intend for something to happen, you are making a request. You want something and so you set your intention. You place the power of your focus on what you want. When you do this, the universe responds immediately. You ask and it answers, every time.

The universe will do all the work for you. It doesn't matter what you want. If you ask for it, it will be given. All you have to do is allow it to be given to you. All you have to do is accept it. You are not a vibrational match to what you want and that's the only reason it does not exist in your reality. You are not a vibrational match to the lean body you want. So, what are you to do? Your body isn't just going to whip itself into shape, is it? That's exactly what it's going to do. You simply have to get out of the way and allow it to find its own balance, on its own schedule. You have to allow your body to receive well-being and return to its natural state.

Your body would be at its optimum weight and size if you were not involved. If you could simply leave your body for a time, it would return to its natural state on its own. It got out of shape because of your habit of thought and your approach to life. You got away from your natural state of well-being, love, and acceptance. Once you return to that state, everything will fall into place.

You created the body you have by choosing to view life from a perspective that has not necessarily served you. That's okay, it happens to many, many people. You may have used food while others may have used alcohol, cigarettes, drugs, sex, video games, TV, gossip, depression, violence, withdrawal, or any other device that could bring some distraction from the emotional stress they were living with. When you return to your natural state of well-being, you will be given the opportunity to remove the habitual reach for something outside yourself to soothe yourself in times of emotional stress. When you learn to do this, you'll stop reaching for foods that don't nourish you, drugs that won't heal you, sex that isn't loving, or anything else that isn't empowering.

Once you begin to listen to what your body is saying, you can keep your focus squarely on your desire. When you feel any negative emotion, whether it's severe or subtle, it is always based in some fear. Realize that the fear isn't real. You are simply making it up. You can't know what's going to happen, so there's no need to use this perspective. Prove the fear is false and choose an empowering perspective and this will make you feel better. There's no need to reach for a snack when you're not hungry. Soothe the fear by proving it's false and choosing to look at it in a way that makes you feel better and then realize that the emotion was fear, not hunger. You don't need to subdue the fear with food; you can reduce the intensity of the fear with rational and thoughtful analysis. This is what will bring your body back into alignment.

Intend to understand that all these little negative emotions that you experience many times a day are caused by fear. Prove the fear is false. Do something that proves it's not real. Don't just sit there and worry; find some evidence that proves you are just making it all up. The fear is your own fabrication. You can make up the fear in your mind and you can also find proof that the fear is false. It is all done in the mind. However, when you act from a low-emotional state of being to ease the fear, now you're bringing it into the physical world. The fear prompts you to take some action to relieve the bad feeling. You might say or do something to harm someone else, or you might say or do something to harm yourself. Actions inspired by thoughts that come from a negative place have the potential to create a reality that you do not want. Therefore, do not take action until you have raised your emotional state and you've returned to feeling good.

When you feel fear, even subtle fear such as boredom, you have dipped ever so slightly into a low emotional state of being. Boredom is a very subtle negative state, but you will still receive inspiration to ease the feeling and so you might be inspired to watch TV, read a gossip magazine, or eat a cookie. These things are done without much awareness of how you are feeling. You are simply looking for a way to distract yourself from your feelings. The action you take from this relatively minor state of being is also minor, but over time it will lead you away from where you want to go.

When you feel hatred, you will be inspired to action that matches the severity of this emotion. You won't receive inspiration to eat a donut, but you might receive inspiration to punch someone. The more intense the negative emotion, the more harmful the action might be. The action taken out of hatred will be one that has the potential to create your reality in a way that you do not want. It will be quite noticeable because the fear is strong. However, even action taken as a result of some minor feeling of stress has the same potential to inspire you to do something that goes against the life you want. So, before taking any action, simply think about your emotional state of being. Are you feeling good or are you feeling bad?

IV.

You have not been taught to analyze your feelings before taking action and so this idea is quite new to you. But it makes sense, doesn't it? You can recall times when you were angry or sad or depressed and you did things you regretted. It was not you; it was the thoughts you attracted due to your low emotional state of being. When you feel bad, you are a match to bad-feeling thoughts. These are the ones that come to you automatically. You could access better-feeling thoughts, but this requires a little concentration. You will instinctually or habitually react with an action inspired from a low-vibrational thought unless you stop and think about it. If you could just stop before reacting, you could find a more empowering thought and you could realize what is happening in the moment.

You have many examples from your own past that illustrate our point. You might have been driving and someone did something that caused you to take offense. You reacted by honking your horn. After you settled down, you might have felt some embarrassment over your reaction and then felt regret. You might have been in a situation where you felt challenged by someone and you were inspired to fight. You might also have thought about it a little and realized that fighting would not solve anything and you backed down. These are examples of action inspired by negative thoughts. You have the ability to think through them and find better-feeling and more empowering thoughts.

When you are inspired to action that comes from a high emotional state of being, such as pride, confidence, happiness, faith, etc., the thoughts that prompt these actions will be in alignment with what you want. The basis of the action will move you toward the creation of the reality you truly want. The action will be empowering. It might not always create the results you want or expect, but the action itself and the idea behind it is completely aligned with your best interests. You can have faith that action inspired from a positive emotional state of being will always be good.

Do not take action when you feel bad. Only take action when you feel good. Intend to feel good and you will be inspired to take action that causes you to feel even better.

This is the most important thing we have to say. Make it your primary intention to feel good and then all thoughts, ideas, words, and actions that are attracted to you will be in complete alignment with who you really are and what you really want. Intend to understand how you really feel in the moment. Intend to understand if the thought you are thinking is empowering or is coming as a result of your lower emotional state. Intend to be a good differentiator of thought. Intend to analyze your thoughts. When you have the thought to eat something, how are you feeling? You see, your urges come as inspiration to act from lower emotional states of being. They are designed to cause you to remove your attention from your emotional distress.

You don't have to be depressed to receive a craving for something that will take your mind off your problems. You could simply be a little anxious. Whatever it is, you are being inspired to do something to take your mind off it. Again, it is your habit to make a change to the outside world. Instead of doing that, you can recognize that the urge is not empowering. It is taking you away from what you really want. It is leading you in a direction away from your desire. Stop and realize what is happening before taking action. Know your emotional state of being.

It is quite different to have a piece of cake while celebrating a birthday than to have a piece of cake to relieve the anxiety of worry. The former is action inspired from a high emotional state of being, while the latter is simply an urge inspired from a negative state. The action taken while celebrating uses the energy of the high emotion and thus well-being continues to flow. That action has no adverse effect on the life experience you truly want. On the other hand, the action taken from the low emotional state uses a negative energy that does contribute to a reality that you do not prefer. The energy is in the emotional state and is transferred to the action. Your emotional state of being powers the action.

Before ordering a meal, think about your emotional state of being. Are you feeling good or bad? If you are feeling good, you will be inspired to order foods that align with feeling good. Conversely, if you are feeling ornery, if you're in a bad mood, if you're brooding over something, stop and think before you order. You know that the first thought will probably resonate with your current state and will not be in harmony with what you truly want. It will be something that will cause you to be distracted from how you are feeling. You can override this urge if you think about it. Thoughts will come, but you can sort through them to find the empowering thoughts and make the better choice in the moment.

V.

If you knew that each and every decision you made was critical to the conscious creation of the life you prefer, you would think more about how you feel before taking action. If you feel good, you will be inspired to action that aligns with how you feel. If you aren't inspired, then no action is required at this time. Isn't that interesting? It turns out that you don't need to be doing something unless you're inspired to do it. If you receive an urge, is that positive inspiration coming from a high-emotional state? Probably not. If you feel excited to do something, is that an urge or inspiration? It's inspiration.

Inspiration is exciting, interesting, and makes sense in the moment. If you're feeling good and you receive inspiration to do something, it will seem logical. It will be as if it's something you simply must do. This action will always be for your greatest benefit and highest good. However, if there is fear involved, you might second guess yourself. If you truly feel inspired, you can overcome the fear and take the action anyway. The feeling you receive from taking action in spite of your fear is exhilaration.

Is every single decision really critical to consciously creating the life you prefer? Of course not. However, when you make decisions after analyzing your emotional state, the decisions will have more of a positive effect on your life. This is what conscious creation is all about. It's the combination of intention, focus, and the analysis of your emotional state. When you understand that thoughts are attracted to you based on your emotional state of being and you can analyze that state, you will understand exactly where the thoughts spring from.

Let's go over a scenario. You wake up in the morning. The new day is always a fresh start. Unless you start thinking about what's been troubling you from yesterday, you will wake in a high-emotional state of well-being. From this state, the decisions you make will be to your benefit. However, most often you immediately start rehashing yesterday's events, troubles, and worries and this causes a dip in your emotional state. So what are you to do? Have a plan. Create a procedure. Start off on the right foot.

We suggest you start your day with an early morning meditation. The meditation will help you quiet your mind. It will set the tone for the new day. Before your meditation, go to the bathroom, drink some water, find a quite place, and set some intentions. Intend that you be able to stop or slow thought. Intend to be mindful and reach a place of ease and well-being. Intend to breathe deeply as you meditate. Intend to be refreshed and renewed. Intend to don the higher perspective. Intend for the meditation to raise your vibration, your energy level, and your mood. Intend for the meditation to create a sense of peace. Intend to feel good.

This is an excellent procedure that, when practiced daily, will help you start each day with the right tone. It will get you feeling good. From this place, you can make your first critical decisions: what to eat for breakfast and what to do for exercise. From this place of feeling good, you will attract thoughts that resonate with how you feel. You want to keep feeling good and so your decisions will be made with the intention of continuing how you feel.

If you could start every day this way, you would quickly and effortlessly make decisions with the intention of continuing to feel good. Remember that how you are feeling today is really the most important consideration. You might worry about how you will feel in the future if you don't get something done today. Try not to think about the future. Keep the focus on now. Keep your decisions short-term. How do you feel now? What can you do now to continue to feel good?

You are accustomed to doing the same things, in the same order, the same way, and the results are usually the same. We want you to think differently now. We want you to do only that which feels good. Think about feeling good. Do you love your work? If so, go to work and enjoy it fully. Do you hate your work? If so, find a way to make the first part of it enjoyable. Don't quit your job just because you hate it. All this will do is cause you to have to find another job and because all you've done was change the outside conditions, the new job will likely be just as bad or even worse than the old one.

If you think you should visit your mother, but she makes you feel bad, then either change the way you allow her to make you feel, or do not visit her. If you feel guilty, realize that this is based on a very limiting belief and that the fear at the base of it is not true. Is it easier for you to ease the feeling of guilt and then not see your mother, or is it easier for you to avoid the guilt by seeing her and then not allowing her to make you feel bad? This is the art of conscious creation. It is always a choice between which decision is most likely to make you feel good in the present moment.

If you find yourself procrastinating, it's because you are not yet inspired to do something. When the inspiration strikes, the timing will be right and you will get the thing done easily. However, if you were to force yourself to do it when the timing is obviously wrong (because you aren't inspired to take action to complete it), then you disengage the forces of the universe and the thing becomes very difficult indeed.

Change your perspective. If there are things you have to do that you do not like, change the way you think about them. Look at it from a more empowering angle. See the benefit of the things you do not like to do. Find something positive in them so that you can feel good about them. This is the work. The work is not to do anything so that in the future you might be happy. The work is to be happy. If there's something you must do, then do it in a way that makes you feel as good as you can about it. If you do not absolutely have to do it, then do not do it.

Chapter Eleven

Become an Allower

Everything you want is coming to you. If you intend to feel good as much and as often as you can, you will enter the state of allowing. What do we mean by that? The state of allowing is one where you are in a place of non-resistance. You do not find anything wrong with the present conditions. You are feeling good. You are going with the flow. You are allowing everything to be as it is. You are not worried. You are not concerned about the future. You have faith that everything is working out for you. You are curious about what will come next. When something happens and you feel negative emotion, you realize it is a manifestation event designed to alter your limiting beliefs and so you do not react negatively to the situation, but rather you approach it with interest and you lean into it.

Everything you want is coming to you. This is the philosophy of a conscious creator. If you want a lean body, then the way to that body is not by doing something drastic like adopting a starvation diet or a painful workout program. The way to receive anything you want, including a lean body, is to allow it to come to you. You can't force it to come. You can't really make it happen. You must allow it to come.

If you try and try and try to make something happen rather than allowing it to come, you fight against the forces of the universe. It is an approach that simply cannot work in an attractive universe. In this reality, you attract that which you desire. Your approach, especially in your Western culture, is to try to effort your way to something. If you don't like the conditions, you work to change them. However, since everything is created from the inside out, if you haven't changed the inside, the outside will always revert back to a reflection of the inside.

When you enter the state of allowing, you are receptive. You put yourself in the mode of receiving. You are attracting by the very creation of your desire and in order for your desire to manifest into your reality, you must receive it. Think of anything you want as a gift. You ask for the gift and you allow the gift to be given. You do not physically create the gift. All you do is birth the desire and expect the universe to bring it to you.

When you have a desire, you become impatient and you want to move the process along by doing something. So you go out and you do it. However, impatience is a low-emotional state of being and from this state you will be given inspiration to act that will counteract the receptive quality needed to allow the gift to be received.

If you desire a lean body, and this is a true desire (meaning you don't want the better-looking body so that you can attract a mate and thereby extinguish your feelings of loneliness), you will be given the lean body you desire. How does the universe give you the lean body you want? It knows that there are several key aspects to shaping your body and it goes to work to put everything in place to create the fullest and most elegant manifestation of your dreams. To accomplish this, the universe must reduce the intensity of your limiting beliefs about yourself and the world around you.

If you were to lose weight by starving yourself and exercising strenuously, you would not have solved the real issue. It's not the weight that is the problem. The weight is the symptom. Your limiting beliefs and your approach to life are the reasons you have the extra weight (and other issues you do not like). Everything stems from your vibration. Your vibration causes weight gain. Raise your vibration and the side effect of that will be the lean body you want as well as everything else you desire.

Let's start by presuming that the only reason you want a lean body is because you think it will feel good. That is the best reason in the world to desire anything. You want the feeling of it. You think it would be nice. You truly, honestly desire a lean body because of the feeling of it and not because you think that the lean body will solve any problem.

So many of you want something because you think that having it will solve some other problem. There is only one way to solve any problem. Realize that it's not a problem, it's simply a message. Understand that you can't solve any problems. You can only work on your vibration. When you see something as a problem, you are making it wrong. Since there is no wrong, only points of view, only limited and higher perspectives, only your bias and individual judgment, you cannot remove the thing to solve the problem. All you can do is change. You can change your perspective, your judgment, and your point of view. You change you, not the thing you do not like.

Back to your body. Do you truly want a lean body because it will be fun, enjoyable, flexible, free, healthy, attractive, and energetic? Then that lean body will be yours. But you have to change. You cannot be the same you and have a lean body. You do not have a lean body, so you must change into the person who does have the body you desire. You aren't doing anything to change your body and you aren't doing anything to change yourself; all you're doing is getting into a receptive mode. All you have to do is become an allower. All you must do is receive anything and everything the universe throws at you.

Let's say you weigh two hundred and fifty pounds and this is seventy pounds more than you would weigh if you had the lean body that was natural for you. Your set of beliefs is perfectly aligned with someone who weighs two hundred and fifty pounds. You are a match to that person in every way. However, you think this weight is wrong and you birth a desire to lose the weight.

Your desire is to lose seventy pounds. Is this a true desire? No. It is a desire that is made to change the conditions in the hopes that the new conditions will make you feel better. You might effort your way to lose the weight, but you'll be fighting the universe the whole way. Instead of receiving inspiration to do things that will cause the changes to be made easily and thus allow the weight to slip away effortlessly, the universe will fight you. You cannot win a fight against the universe.

Since you are focused on how wrong your weight is, the universe brings you urges and cravings and pain and thoughts of other things. It wants you to be the weight you are now. It doesn't want you to lose a pound. Why is the universe fighting you and keeping you where you are? Because that's where your focus is. All of your attention is placed on the weight. All you are thinking about is how wrong the weight is. The universe can only see what you are focusing your attention on. You are shining a light on your weight, so the universe assumes that you are asking for more weight. Every thought you receive is designed to help you keep the weight on.

We understand your frustration and confusion. You must think the universe is crazy. Why would anyone want to keep weight on? There must be a flaw in the system. Shouldn't I simply focus on what I don't like and have that removed? That would be so much easier. Well, if this is what you are thinking, there's a flaw in your premise.

If you looked at things you did not like and you could obliterate them out of existence, then there would be no Earth. Man would have already wiped out that which they did not want and therefore nothing would exist. It's nearly happened many times before, but the universe has always intervened because the system was designed to be creative, not destructive. You can create anything you like, but you cannot destroy anything. When you believe you have eradicated something, this is an illusion. Nothing can be completely destroyed unless it wants to be.

So give up this approach. Stop trying to change the conditions. Stop thinking about pushing things away. Start realizing that you can't run away from things you don't like. You cannot hide. You can only focus on what is wanted and leave everything else alone. It is all good. It is all right. There is no wrong. Turn the other cheek toward what you want and allow that to come to you. This is the approach to life that will yield the greatest results and the most enhanced life experience. Set an intention to become an allower.

II.

Allowing is natural. In a natural world, free from the influences of your fearful society, you would live a life of ease, conjuring up one desire after another and expecting those desires to manifest in the most elegant manner imaginable. Your life would be one of ease, acceptance, unconditional love, and complete freedom. You could have, be, and do anything you dreamed of. It would be paradise.

This is not the life you are living now. Your life is fraught with worry, anxiety, fear, and lack. You think you must work to get things done. You think you must be continually doing. You think money will solve your problems and so you slave away your lives doing things you do not enjoy, just to scratch together a little money that does little to ease your worries.

We want to tell you that there is a better way. There is an approach to life that is not defined by what you are doing, but rather by how you are being. Being is a state based in the present moment. How you are being will create what unfolds in your future. If you are being worried in this moment, you will resonate with those things you are worried about. If you are being trusting, you will resonate with that which you hope for.

Being creates your present state. Your emotional state of being is the vibration that you are emitting. Everything responds to how you are being. When you are being calm, you are in a receiving mode. When you are being stressed, you are in a resistant mode. The key to creating the reality you desire is to be in the nonresistant state of being known as allowing.

Imagine that your state of being either draws in that which you want or keeps it away. You are either being receptive or repulsive. When you are being receptive, that which you want comes easily. When you are being repulsive, that which you want seems as if it is being kept from you. In reality, you cannot repulse anything; however, you can and do create the illusion that what you really want is not within your reach.

Everything you want exists now. The lean body you want is within easy reach. It's just that you cannot see it. From your present state of being, it appears that the body you so desire does not exist. Instead, all you see is the body you do not want. How is this possible? How can the body you do not want exist in place of the body you do want, even when the lean body you desire is so easily within reach? It is simply an illusion caused by your present state of being.

Who you are being now cannot see how to easily get to where you want to go. You have created the illusion of difficulty. This is an extremely important concept to grasp. You are being fooled into thinking that the thing you want is not available to you right now. If you could shift your perception just a little, all the answers would be revealed to you and you would have anything you desired, instantly.

Let's examine this a bit further. You see yourself as overweight and you would like to actually, physically be thinner. You would like to have less fat, more muscle, and look better. You would like to feel better in your body. We tell you that the lean body you want exists right now and that you cannot see it because you have a perceptual issue that creates the illusion that you are overweight. Does this make any sense at all? Let's look at an example.

You know of people who experience the condition known as anorexia nervosa. These people have a perception of themselves as being overweight, so they try to offset this perception by losing weight. However, they were never overweight to begin with. They simply see themselves as fat and they are desperate to remove the fat. It's not that they are actually fat, it's only that they perceive themselves to be fat. With proper treatment and care, they can eventually alter their perception of themselves so that they can once again see themselves as normal and healthy.

If you were living in a society where everyone was fat, it would feel normal to be fat. You may not like it, but you would not think so badly of it. In fact, many of you became overweight because you were not exposed to too much judgment against your excess weight. However, you all have some degree of perceptual dissonance. Your perception of what is right is different than how you see yourself. You are seeing yourself as wrong. Like the anorexics, you are looking in the mirror and judging yourself to be less than adequate and this causes inner conflict. The more you see yourself as wrong, the more often you create your state of being as wrong. From this state, you create. You create your reality based on your state of being. If you are living in the state of being of one who perceives himself or herself as fat, you are creating your reality based on this perception.

If you could shift your perception from one who thinks of himself as fat to one who thinks of himself as lean, then you would instantly begin creating that. The shift would occur instantaneously. As soon as you saw yourself as lean, you would be lean and you would create from this perspective of yourself.

Everyone who is lean thinks of himself as a lean person unless they have some mental/perceptual condition. Everyone who thinks of himself as fat is fat to the degree or their perception. The question now becomes one of altering perception.

If you perceive yourself to be lean, you are lean. If you perceive yourself to be fat, you are fat. If you have the lean perception and someone calls you fat, you can't really hear that. It doesn't resonate with you. You won't internalize the statement. At worst you might consider that you have put on a pound or two and you'll allow it to be removed easily. You'll be inspired to do something that makes you feel good and the weight will come right off. For the lean person, this is not only easy to do, it's fun, challenging, and rewarding.

If you perceive yourself to be fat and someone compliments you on how you look, you'll wave it off or give credit to some other factor, such as your hair, clothes, lighting, make-up, or that they were being nice and didn't really mean it. Your perception creates your reality. You perceive yourself as overweight and so you are the version of yourself that is overweight. You behave, eat, act, and think like one who is overweight. Everything you think, say, and do resonates with one who is overweight. But this is just perception. It is not truth.

The truth has nothing to do with the perception. The perception is false unless it serves you. You can perceive anything as you want it to be. Perception is in the eyes of the perceiver. You can alter your perception. You can alter your state of being. You can be different. You can think differently. You can have anything you want if you will just alter your perception slightly. It is all within reach. It all has to do with your thoughts, not with what is reflected back to you by the mirror of your current reality.

III.

The state of allowing is entered through the doorway of acceptance. Unconditional love is unconditional acceptance. Who you really are is a being of unconditional love. Who you really are is one who accepts everything unconditionally. If you are not accepting, you are not allowing. If you are accepting, you are receiving. If you are resistant, you are not allowing, accepting, or receiving. In order to receive something, you must somehow enter the state of allowing.

When you look at something and judge it as wrong, you are simply choosing to resist what is. There is no wrong anywhere in the universe. Everything is right. If it exists in your reality, it is a vibrational match to who you are being and therefore it is right and necessary. It cannot be any other way. If you decide that it is wrong, that it should not exist, that you don't like it, then you are simply arguing with your own creation.

Everything that exists in your life is your creation and it is all good. If it's something that you don't prefer, then ignore it. Give no attention to it. Walk around it. Do not try to destroy it; just leave it be and find something else. Someone else might like it.

When something pops up in your life, it is there for you even when you don't think it is. If it came, it came as a response to your vibration. Everything you want is coming to you. You must be transformed in order for you to see it. Sometimes you hold onto some very limiting beliefs and these thought forms create the illusion that what you want is out of your reach. When you can shift your perception by altering the intensity of these limiting beliefs, suddenly the illusion is removed.

If you had no limiting beliefs, everything you wanted would come to you rather quickly and easily. You would have no resistance and therefore your vibration would easily match whatever you desired and the desire would manifest. You would be able to alter your perception on your own. Your limiting beliefs are like the lock on the desire. Your ability to alter your perception is the key.

If you could see your limiting beliefs, you could analyze each one and reduce their intensity on your own. You could find proof that each limiting belief is false. You could do this during meditation and as you emerged from your meditative state, your perception would be altered and your reality would shift to something new. However, you do not understand that you could or should analyze your own limiting beliefs. You don't know what it means. You can't know the tremendous benefit. You cling to your limitations like they are a suit of armor.

When you accept the conditions as they are, you are agreeing with the design of the universe. You understand that the conditions have been created to support whatever it is you came here to explore. You know that your body is part of that exploration and that it is perfect as it is because it is allowing you to explore reality in the way you intended. If you look at any aspect of it and think it's inadequate, then you cannot trust that this is all for you. You are either a conscious creator and believe that this is all part of the process of expansion and growth and you take responsibility for your creation, or you must perceive yourself as a victim without any responsibility.

When you decide to perceive yourself as a creator and you've created a condition you do not like, you must also accept that your creation is perfect and that you are a masterful creator. This seems like a paradox. If you are a conscious creator, and you created something that exists in your reality but you realize that it is something you do not like, how can you possibly see it as perfect? You must see it as perfect because the creation is part of your expansion and all expansion is good. You came here for expansion and you also knew that you could expand in joy. It's simply how you perceive the condition that causes you to believe you are an inferior creator.

If you are overweight, the weight is a symptom of something else. The weight is your catalyst to move through something you are resisting. Without the weight, you would have no way to understand the issue you need to resolve. You came here to explore and maybe even to conquer this issue. The symptom lets you know that you are resisting this exploration and as a result you are feeling inner conflict. The irritation of this inner conflict (a nagging feeling) needs to be resolved. You can resolve it by tackling it head on or you can soothe yourself by eating, drinking, smoking or any other distraction. But the use of outside devices to distract from inner feelings builds momentum and leads to unwanted exterior conditions. Your outer reality reflects your inner reality.

If you have a health problem, a financial issue, an addiction, or any other unwanted condition, it all stems from resistance to some aspect of your life that you willingly and intentionally came here to explore. By attempting to remove the inner feeling with an outer action, you create dissonance. You are simply attempting to avoid the thing by calling it wrong.

You were born into a family that you specifically chose because you knew the environment of your youth would set you on a course to explore certain aspects of physical reality. The conditions of your childhood were perfectly designed for you. When you look back and criticize something in your childhood, you are arguing with the perfection of the universe and the wisdom of your intentions. When you believe that some aspect of it was wrong or bad, you deny the creative qualities of that specific childhood that gave you the wonderful opportunity and incentive to create the life you live today.

You might be able to look back at your childhood and remember how comfortable it was most of the time. You might remember the families of your friends and how different their families were. It felt different in their homes. Some more loving and others less so. However, you were a match to your family and they were a match to theirs. You would most likely feel uncomfortable living in another family because you were not a match to another family. Of course, there are always exceptions and if this is the case then you actually were a vibrational match to another family and this too was part of the trajectory you intended. You chose it all; the good and everything you still think was bad.

If you could see your life from the higher perspective, you would understand that everything has been and is working out perfectly. You would not exchange the difficult parts of your life, because they led you to where you are now. When you look back with regret or resentment, you are simply resisting the trajectory you chose. In reality, it was all perfect. The only problem was your resistance to a lot of it. Had you known that you were resisting, you might have allowed it to come easier than it did. But, that too, is part of the process.

You could not pick up this book and read it this far if you were not a vibrational match to much of the information contained within these pages. You cannot assimilate all of the information we are presenting because no one is a match to all of it. But you are coming to understand much of what we are teaching. You are interested and receptive and as you read this book, your vibration is rising. As you raise your vibration, you become more receptive and are able to internalize more and more information that now resonates with your new vibrational level.

When you view something as wrong, out of place, or inconsistent with what you want, you are resisting it. It is not wrong for you; it only seems wrong. You think you don't want it, but all you are doing is resisting it. If you gave up your resistance, the thing would present its message to you and then leave your reality because it is no longer necessary.

Let's look at another example. This is the most common of examples and it is the limiting belief that you are not worthy. Everyone on Earth has this belief to a degree and it is the most limiting and most false of all the limiting beliefs in existence. As a child, you were told you were wrong. You were punished for doing something that your parents, teachers, society, or even your peers judged as wrong. In fact, you did nothing wrong; you were simply caught up in the act of exploration. However, they judged it as bad behavior and they chose to correct the behavior by making you wrong.

You felt as if you were wrong or they were wrong. To you it seemed as if they loved you a bit less than before. You may have attempted to modify your behavior in order to regain their love. From this point on you played a role. The role was either a rebel who refused to kneel to their demands or one who altered their behavior in order to behave in a way that would allow the flow of love to continue. You sought their approval and in doing so you became an altered version of yourself. You could not be your authentic self.

This caused a pattern and momentum was started. You began behaving in ways that were acceptable to your parents, teachers, friends, and society. You started judging the behavior of others, and those who dropped outside the lines of decent behavior were judged harshly. In doing so you lost track of who you really are and this caused a feeling of dissonance. You were not resonating with who you really are. There was a chasm between the two realities; who you really are versus who you are being.

You could realign yourself with who you really are on your own. You could recognize that your parents, teachers, peers, and society were all operating in fear. All of their actions and judgments were based in fear. They forced you to adopt their fears. One fear created the next and was handed down the family line. You received some of the fears adopted by generations who came before you, even though these fears need not exist in your life.

You were born with the knowledge that you are worthy, but somewhere along the line you adopted the belief that you were not completely worthy. You tried to alter that by doing the only thing you knew how to do: you tried to change the outside conditions so that you could feel better. The conditions cannot be physically changed because they are created from within in a nonphysical way. You try and try and try to get others to love you by doing all the things you think they want you to do. You are nice, you are friendly, you might go to church, or get good grades, or make money, or bring home flowers. You pay your bills on time and you conform to dress codes, moral codes, and all other standards of behavior. But one thing is missing. You are not being you and so you feel discontent.

The discontent is mild, yet it is palpable. You are used to it, but it is always there. Sometimes you get tired of faking it and you throw a temper tantrum to express yourself. You don't know what's wrong, so you soothe yourself in any way you can. You are avoiding the issue mostly because you are unaware it exists.

People are trying to change you and you are yielding to their wishes. You are wanting them to change as well. Instead of being who you are, doing what you want, and having all that you desire, you limit yourself in order to receive the approval, the recognition, and the acceptance of others. This, however, cannot work. You didn't come here to please others; you came for your personal expansion and growth.

You are playing a game of tug and war. You are being who you are not to gain love, just like you were taught as a child, and you are also wanting to express yourself and live life on your terms. This isn't a bad thing, it's just that you are resisting a lot of it.

When something pops up that confronts your false impression of you, which is the reason it pops up, you resist it. You stick to your limitations. You hold on tightly to your false beliefs. You refuse to acknowledge that there might be a better way. It seems painful, so you hide from it.

Instead, we ask you to lean in. If something appears painful, lean into it rather than running away from it. Realize that it is there for you. Understand that you have nothing to fear. Seek the information contained in it. Allow it to alter your beliefs about yourself. You are not being who you are and until you drop your facade, you will always encounter painful moments because you will always resist them. Resistance is the only thing that causes pain. It's never the thing itself; it's only how you are choosing to look at the thing.

IV.

Pain is self-inflicted. You shy away from situations that might give rise to negative emotion because you fear the pain associated with these emotions. In doing so, you are not confronting the issue at hand. In order to get what you truly want, in order to live life on your terms, you must move through the issue that presents itself. You must walk through the burning coals. If you have seen the fire walk where people walk on burning coals with their bare feet, you can see how they literally move through their fear. When they find themselves on the other side without burns on their feet, they feel exhilaration. It looked scary, but they moved through their fear and emerged not only unscathed, but also vibrationally elevated. The process of moving through fear is an act that causes a raising of vibration.

You find yourself placed in a situation that causes some fear. Instead of dealing with the situation (walking through the hot coals), you back down from it and avoid it. There really is nothing to fear; you simply perceive it to be scarier than it really is. If it is presented in your life, it is there for a reason. It could not be there otherwise. If you simply entered the situation with love, acceptance, and an understanding that it was for your benefit, you would emerge from the other side in a much better place. Your vibration would be raised and your reality would shift to reflect your newer, higher vibration. Things would be better.

When you hide from these issues (the issues you specifically came here to explore) because you fear the emotion that might come up, you are resisting life. In doing so, you restrict your own growth and expansion. This resistance causes stress. In order to relieve the stress, you suppress your feelings by eating, drinking, or some other distraction. If you are overweight, you are suppressing your feelings with food. If you are drinking in excess, you are suppressing uncomfortable feelings with alcohol. If you are doing drugs, you are suppressing your feelings with drugs. If you are addicted to any outside distraction, it's because you are suppressing the feelings caused by resistance. The side effect of suppressed feelings is weight gain, alcohol and drug abuse, sex addiction, illness, etc.

You choose to suppress your emotions for one reason and one reason only; you fear the negative emotion. You hate the feeling of negative emotion. You attempt to control the external conditions because you are afraid of feeling any negative emotion. Fear causes you to seek conditions that are safe and pleasant. When you do this, you are avoiding the aspects of physical reality that you came to explore. This avoidance creates stress and to deal with the stress, you turn to some distraction. And often, as a result, you develop a condition called weight gain, addiction, illness, etc.

When you become an allower, you drop your fear of negative emotion. In fact, you embrace negative emotion because you know that an opportunity for growth and expansion is presenting itself. The only reason negative emotion could arise within you is due to an issue that is being presented to you. You must accept the emotion as a sign that something special is happening. You have some limiting belief based in an irrational fear and you must confront it. Why do you feel bad? What is the fear? Are you going to analyze it or will you judge the whole story to be wrong?

A person who resists these manifestation events and does not see the benefit in them will not push through them. You will not grow into the version of you who is ready for your dreams to manifest in your reality.

If you are overweight and you want to lose the weight, you must allow the transformation you have asked for to take place. The only way you can transform from who you are now to the person who is ready for your desire to unfold is to move through these manifestation events, despite the painful feeling of negative emotion.

As an allower, you will face many manifestation events, but as a person who resists, you will run away from these manifestation events. The events are for your growth. They are designed to reduce the intensity of limiting beliefs. If you resist them, you will not be able to create the lean body you want. Use your weight loss goals as motivation for growth. Know that shying away from unpleasant-feeling emotions will not enable you to lose weight because you will not be resolving the issues that caused the weight to be gained in the first place. Your weight is a side effect of the stress created by unresolved issues.

The concept that there is no wrong anywhere in the universe is what allowing is all about. If there is no wrong, there is no resistance. If you perceive everything as right, you are an allower. Without resistance, you can move easily from the vibration you are emitting right now, which is creating the life you are currently living, to a new and higher vibration that will create the life you prefer.

Your desire creates the need to alter your vibration. If you had no desires, if you were perfectly content, you would feel no resistance. You would experience no negative emotion. However, since you have birthed a desire, the universe is answering your request. You do not match whatever it is you want and therefore you must be changed. If your desire is to come to you, you must become a match to it. It's as simple as that. If you allow the changes to your beliefs to be made, you will easily become a match to that which you want. If you resist any change to your belief system, you will feel negative emotion. The negative emotion need not be painful; it's simply a message letting you know that you are resisting the change you want. If you can release your limiting beliefs, you will remove the barrier that separates you from your desire. That is all that is going on here.

Allowing is the acknowledgment that everything that shows up in your life is for your benefit, whether it seems like it or not. You might judge it as bad, but that is just resistance. It is good. If you can see it as progress toward that which you want, then you are an allower. If you choose to hang on to your limiting beliefs and suffer through the negative emotion that comes with resistance, then that too is your choice. Chose to allow limiting beliefs to fade and you will receive all that you want. Resist any challenge to your limiting beliefs and not only will you prevent your desire from being manifested in your reality, but you'll also experience continued negative emotion.

V.

Imagine that your desire was to create a healthy, lean body that felt good. This is not only possible, but perfectly natural. Your body's natural state is healthy and lean. Any deviation from perfect health and a body that feels good is brought on by consistently resisting that which challenges the negative beliefs that keep you apart from everything you desire. If you had no limiting beliefs, you would encounter no resistance and your dreams would manifest one after another. However, you are used to thinking in a way that keeps whatever you want from coming into your life. It doesn't matter what it is. If you desire a mate and that mate has eluded you, it's due to one or more limiting beliefs. Those beliefs will be challenged until you either alter your beliefs or give up your desire. It is simply the mechanism of physical reality.

When your beliefs are challenged through a manifestation event, you will feel discord in the form of negative emotion. You might feel sad, discouraged, shame, bitterness, envy, jealousy, etc. All of these negative emotions are designed to wake you up to the fact that you are looking at the subject in a way that does not serve you. Your perspective is flawed and unless you adopt a new perspective and a more empowering set of beliefs, you will not be able to manifest the relationship you desire.

This is may be a difficult concept to understand. You believe there is some valid reason that you cannot create the relationship you so desire. This is not true. There is no valid reason. The relationship you want is there; you just can't see it. It is an illusion. The belief that you hold onto that prevents you from discovering the relationship is simply false. You believe it to be true, but this belief is limiting and therefore it is absolutely false. If you can see that it is not true, that it is based on an irrational fear, you can reduce its effect on your life. It does not have to affect you. It can be dealt with.

No one is going to help you but you. It's up to you to discover how the universe works, how your beliefs work, and how you can alter them through the art of analysis. There is no true support group. Most people you know are committed to the old approach to life. This approach, where you make things happen and you ignore negative emotion, does not work. They will counsel you and persuade you to keep trying what is not working; however, you have found a new approach.

The new approach to life is one of allowing, not pushing against. It is one of receiving, not taking. It is one of patience, not performance. In this approach to life, you focus your power of attention on what you prefer and how you feel. This is a feeling reality and the only thing that really matters is how you feel. Do you feel good? Then that is what matters. Are you experiencing negative emotion? Then stop and analyze the fear at the basis of the limiting belief and find a new, higher perspective that creates the feeling of relief.

In the new approach to life, your goal is to feel good now, not some time in the future when your dream manifests into your reality. Feel good now and you create an environment where your dreams can manifest. It doesn't matter if you're going to feel good in the future unless you can feel good in the present moment. Don't do anything unless it feels good now. If it isn't fun, interesting, or enjoyable, don't do it. Do things that are appealing or wait for inspiration to strike.

When you are focused on feeling good, inspiration is always striking. You receive thoughts and when you follow them, they will lead to people, places, and events that will move you toward that which you desire. These thoughts may lead you right into a manifestation event that will challenge your beliefs. This could be painful if you resist it, but when you understand what's going on, there's no need for emotional pain or resistance. This is a chance to alter some of your limiting beliefs. Once you've done that, you are another step closer to realizing a dream.

Back to the diet. Let's talk about this from the perspective of an allower. You feel overweight, bloated, unattractive, and lethargic. You want to feel good. You believe that losing weight will make you feel better. You think about how nice it will feel to have more energy, look better, and be healthier. So you create the very strong desire to become the lean and healthy person you naturally are. The universe hears your request and immediately goes to work.

If you knew nothing about how the universe works, and you created the desire to lose weight but you also paid attention to how fat you currently are, then you've created your own tug of war. On the one hand, the universe is working on your desire to lose weight by placing you in situations that challenge your limiting beliefs, and on the other hand, the universe is sending you urges designed to keep the weight on because you are paying so much attention to your current weight. This paradox is the reason the vast majority of those who attempt to lose weight ultimately fail.

How can you lose weight and keep it off when you do not understand the mechanism of physical reality? When you are unaware of the most fundamental laws of the universe, you have little chance of manifesting that which you want when you are focused on what is not wanted. The manifestation process, given your resistant approach to life, becomes quite difficult indeed. In order to become a successful manifestor, you must become an allower.

The first step is to create your desire. You do not need to formalize it; it is completely developed internally and is articulated through your vibration. Your words could not adequately describe the intricacies of your desire. Once it is born, it is out there and the universe receives it immediately. This is the second step.

The third step in the manifestation process is for you to allow it to come. This part is completely up to you. You can change your mind at any time and the manifestation process will be halted. You can continue to focus on the absence of your desire and the process will be stalled. You can resist the changes that must be made and again the process is stalled. It is easier for you to resist the process than it is to allow it. Allowing takes some focus, practice, and patience.

If you are an allower, you know that focusing on your present weight and noticing that you do not like what you see in the mirror is detrimental to the manifestation process. As an allower, you choose to recognize that your body is perfect as it is. You are not results-oriented. To be focused on results means that you will choose to feel good when the desired results have been achieved. This again is the old approach to life. You must choose to feel good now, results be damned. You choose to accept the conditions of your body and your life as they exist now as perfect, because that's exactly what they are. They cannot be different than they are in the moment, so they must be considered perfect. They are the perfect representation of your current vibration. Change your vibration and you will receive a new set of perfect conditions that perfectly match your new vibration. That's how the system works.

As an allower, you recognize that your body and all aspects of your life are perfect. You appreciate the good parts and the parts you judge as not so good. It must be considered all good. You have preferences and your desires are created based on these preferences. That's good. You do not need to do anything else. You do not have to condemn the things you do not prefer. If you prefer being lean, that is wonderful, but it does not mean that being anything other than lean is bad or wrong.

When you get to a place of acceptance of what is, you create an environment of allowing. In this environment, your dreams have fertile ground in which to grow and develop. Without this environment, your dreams will not manifest. Every single desire that manifested in your reality started coming as soon as you created an environment of allowing. Even if you did not know what you were doing, you somehow figured out a way to create that allowing environment.

You accept the size and shape of your body as perfect in this moment. It is the perfect place to start. This is about much more than losing a little weight. This is about the creation of the life you prefer in all areas. This goal of weight loss is a metaphor for everything you want. You can create anything using the same process. If you can lose some weight and create the lean and healthy body you desire, you can also create the relationships of your dreams, the abundance of your dreams, and everything else you want. It all starts with creating the environment of allowing by seeing everything as perfect as it is.

Your body is perfect and this time and place is perfect. You are not yet a match to a lean body. In order to become a match, you must change your vibration so that your vibration reflects the reality of a lean and healthy person. If you were a lean and healthy person right now, you would have a vibration that emitted the signal of a lean and healthy person. Your vibration emits a different signal. Why is that?

Your vibration is comprised basically of the thoughts you think. There is certainly more to it than that, but for now, this is the basic information that you must understand. Your beliefs are strong and intense thought forms. All of your thoughts align with your beliefs. Your beliefs are made more powerful by the Law of Attraction. What you believe is reflected back to you by the reality you witness with your physical senses. When your beliefs are challenged, you feel negative emotion and it is your habit to hold on tightly to your beliefs. This is fine when your beliefs are beneficial; however, when your beliefs are limiting, when they hold you apart from your dreams, then they do not serve you and they are not true.

If not for your limiting beliefs and your attitude about life, you would easily manifest everything you truly desire. If you could simply turn off each limiting belief, one by one, you would see a dramatic shift in the quality of your life. However, you cannot completely turn off a limiting belief. They can only be dimmed. Once a belief exists, it exists eternally. The intensity of the belief can be modified and that is a very good thing. You can reduce the intensity of limiting beliefs by proving they are false and you can raise the intensity of beneficial beliefs by proving they are true. This is how you adjust your vibration so it comes within the frequency range of what you really want.

You could adjust your vibration yourself or you could allow the universe to do it for you. It's your choice. It might be easier just to let the universe do it. After all, you aren't even aware of most of your limiting beliefs. You don't even recognize that they are limiting. If you sat down to write a list of your limiting beliefs, you would not think of very many. The universe knows exactly which beliefs limit which desires. It will place you in situations designed to flush out your limiting beliefs. These are called manifestation events. Whenever you feel negative emotion, you are in a manifestation event.

The negative emotion is your clue that 1) you're in a manifestation event, and 2) you have a limiting belief that needs to be altered. The problem with this wonderful process is your relationship with negative emotion. You are either so used to feeling negative emotion that the feeling doesn't signify anything to you because you're numb to it, or you find it so traumatic that you shy away from any situation that has the potential to cause negative emotion. Unless you understand the purpose of the emotion, you have little chance of analyzing your limiting beliefs and then reducing their intensity.

Most people go into a manifestation event blind. They don't know what's happening; all they know is that they feel bad. They look to blame someone or something outside of themselves and they try to solve the emotion by judging the conditions of the event as wrong. They might believe that it was not their fault that this happened, that it was a random act of fate. They do not understand that the manifestation was their creation (at least partly) and that it exists to serve them by exposing one or more limiting beliefs. Even when conscious creators analyze recent manifestation events, they often have difficulty identifying the limiting beliefs. It seems difficult only because you're just now learning the rules of the game. It is new to you. Had you been educated on this process from birth, you would be masters at recognizing limiting beliefs.

Every single person on the planet has a set of limiting beliefs, some more than others. Your set of limiting beliefs is unique to you as is everything else about your existence. Your perspective is unique. What works for others may or may not work for you. There's no way to tell unless you experiment.

Chapter Twelve

Experimentation

You are a unique physical being. What works for others only works for them because they have found something that is a match to their unique vibration. What doesn't work for others is only because they have not aligned with the vibration of it. It has nothing to do with anything other than vibration. You are either a vibrational match to something or you are not.

When you hear about a new diet and how it's worked for many people, what is happening is a mass shift of beliefs. People who believe that something is working temporarily enter the state of allowing and come into vibration range of the thing they want. They use their belief in this new diet to cause themselves to suspend their limiting beliefs, if only for a little while. And it works as long as their limiting beliefs remain low in intensity. However, as soon as their limiting beliefs come back, their weight returns.

Healing works in a similar fashion. One drug may work for one person and not another. What's the difference? Their unique vibrations. A person's vibration is the sum of their feelings, beliefs, attitudes, approach to life, and the thoughts they consistently think. Every person is different. One person may allow themselves to be healed by a drug, while another person remains doubtful. Everyone is different, even though each dose of a drug has the same vibration. It is the interaction between the drug's vibration and the person's vibration that either aligns or not.

If you want a diet to work for you, you must come into vibrational alignment with that diet. The diet isn't perfect for you unless you adjust your vibration to reach the vicinity of the diet's vibration. The diet is nonphysical. It is just an idea. It is a thought form. It is a method based on believability. You could adopt any diet and either lose weight or gain weight depending on your belief system. If you can adjust your beliefs to match the idea of the diet, then the diet will work for you, as long as your beliefs are a match to the idea. As soon as something happens to shake your confidence in the diet (or your ability to achieve results you believe are appropriate) the intensity of your limiting beliefs begins to rise and the diet no longer works for you. This is the cause of yo-yo dieting.

When you are excited by the potential of a new diet, you suspend your limiting beliefs about yourself and allow what you want to enter your reality. In this case, you allow the weight to fall off because you believe the diet will work. As long as you are seeing positive results, your limiting beliefs are reduced in intensity enough for you to allow the weight loss to occur. At some point you will reengage those limiting beliefs and notice that the diet no longer works. Your vibration will return to the same place it was before and your reality will shift to match it. You'll regain the weight and maybe a bit more.

This becomes a cycle of weight loss when limiting beliefs are lowered and weight gain when they return to their previous intensity. The beliefs may be about anything. You might have a limiting belief that you cannot be thin. You might believe that you cannot be loved, or successful, or happy, or grateful, or forgiving, or nice, or any one of a thousand things. You may be holding onto regret or resentment. You may be suppressing feelings of anger. Whatever the limiting beliefs are, the diet temporarily lowers their intensity long enough for you to lose some weight, but eventually the limiting beliefs rise back to the surface and your body reverts back to where it was before you found the diet.

The same thing will happen with this diet. Our diet is no different. We are presenting you with an idea. If you believe in this idea, you will suppress your limiting beliefs for a while. The longer you suppress your limiting beliefs, the more success you will have. However, if you do not also radically change your approach to life, then eventually your old beliefs will reemerge and your reality will shift to match your old vibration.

Your weight has nothing to do with anything other than your vibration. Your vibration is the sum of your feelings, beliefs, attitudes, approach to life, and the thoughts you consistently think. Change your vibration temporarily and your world will temporarily shift to match your vibration. In order to permanently change your reality, you must make a permanent change to your vibration.

Anyone can temporarily change their vibration. You do it all the time. When you are in a good mood, your reality matches your mood. When you are in a bad mood, the same thing happens. Your reality shifts as easily and as often as your mood changes. However, permanent change requires a complete change in your perspective. The way you look at the world around you must be different if you are to receive a different reality.

Your vibration will shift as a result of this book, and for many people that alone will create an improvement in their life. The degree to which their lives improve will correlate with how much they changed their vibration as a result of reading this book. It is an interesting thing. You come to this book with a set of beliefs both beneficial and limiting. By the end of this book your core beliefs will be changed. You will see life from a higher and broader perspective and your life will change as a result.

Some people will read this book and resonate with certain concepts. Everything we are saying will resonate with you if you allow it to. However, you have some beliefs that will be in conflict with some of what we have to say and on these subjects you will either not change your beliefs, not understand what we are really saying, or skip over them entirely. But if you read this entire book cover to cover, you will be changed by it. Your vibration will rise and you will see things from a new perspective.

If you read this book, you will receive new thoughts and ideas as a result. You will be led to other books, other topics of interest, and new ideas will come to you. This is due to your new, higher vibration. When you reread this book from a higher vibrational level, you will encounter new words and ideas that you had completely missed your first time through. That is because you are now a vibrational match to more ideas contained in this book. Each time your vibration rises, you become a match to new ideas and thoughts.

II.

If you permanently alter the intensity of a limiting belief, your life will permanently change to reflect your new vibrational signal. We shouldn't use the word "permanent" because you are always changing and shifting, but we are saying that the apparent change in your reality will now reflect the frequency of your new vibration as a result of your new system of beliefs. Change one belief and your life also changes. Adopt a new limiting belief and your life becomes more limited. Reduce the intensity of a limiting belief and your life becomes less limited.

You might have a belief that exercise is painful, uncomfortable, time-consuming, and unpleasant. This is a limiting belief for you. Your reality reflects this belief to the degree to which you believe it to be true. If you hate any form of exercise, you experience a reality where exercise is unpleasant. While this is true for you, can you see that it is not true for many, many people? By recognizing that what applies to you does not apply to other people, you have just reduced the intensity of a very limiting belief.

Let's say you have the limiting belief that physical activity is painful, tiring, and unpleasant. When you exercise, you feel uncomfortable. It isn't fun. When you look at others exercising, you imagine that they are all simply pushing through the pain. Your limiting belief about exercise is just about as intense as it gets. Now, how do you intentionally go about reducing the intensity of this belief that is obviously limiting your experience of life? You prove to yourself that it is false.

Physical activity is painful. This is your belief. Is it true? You might answer yes to this question. In your experience, exercise is painful. Now ask yourself if this is always true. It isn't. When you walk, it is not painful. There are occasions when you are doing something fun where pain is not a factor. By noticing these examples where your belief is not always true, and ny proving that fact to yourself by bringing up examples in your own experience, you diminish the intensity of your limiting belief and your world adjusts slightly to reflect your new overall set of beliefs.

Physical exercise is not enjoyable. This is another limiting belief, but you just provided yourself with evidence that proves this belief is false as well. People play sports and this is fun for them. Have you ever played sports for fun? If so, this is proof that the limiting belief is false. By acknowledging that your belief is false, you reduce its intensity. Now it's time to experiment.

Experimentation

You previously believed that physical activity was painful and was not fun. You showed yourself evidence that your beliefs were false and this reduced the intensity of those beliefs. However, they still exist and they remain intense enough that they affect your reality. To reduce them further, you must have personal experience that denies the very existence of the belief. When you use personal experience to prove a belief is false, you diminish its intensity so that it no longer has the power to affect your life. You must think of some form of physical activity that is both fun and pain-free. What will you come up with?

Here is where inspiration plays a role. From a positive emotional state of being, you think about all the forms of physical activity that might be both painless and fun. Soon thoughts will enter your head. You will think about them and try to imagine if they would be appropriate for you. As soon as an inspiring thought comes into your mind, you might also feel fear. What if it isn't fun? What if it is painful? What if this is not a good idea? What if I can't do it? What if people make fun of me for the way I look? What if I don't fit in? What if it's too expensive? The same fears that kept you from doing physical activity in the first place pop up the moment you receive inspiration to act. These fears are all irrational and are all false. You must continue your work to prove that they are false as well.

This is what experimentation is all about. Experimentation is a device that will alleviate your irrational fears. You have an inspiration to do some form of physical activity that is fun and painless. You are inspired to play golf, for instance. You have never played golf before and you receive many fearful thoughts. Without the device of experimentation, you would succumb to your fears. You would never try anything. However, the device we call experimentation allows you to suppress your fears and try the activity that has been inspired.

A fear might arise, such as "What if it isn't fun?" You can now answer that question by saying, "I don't know if it will be fun, but I am willing to experiment to find out." Because it is just an experiment and not a commitment, you are free to try out your inspired activity without allowing the fear to disrupt the activity. You have little invested and this alleviates the fear. You can use the experimentation device on any fear. "I have a fear and I am going to try this experiment to see if the fear is true."

The more you are open to the idea of experimentation, the more you will find it easier to dismiss your fears. Fear arises at the moment of inspiration because you start to think of all the things that could go wrong. You believe in the possibility of failure. There is no failure, there is only experience and all experience is valid and valuable. If you think to yourself, "This is just an experiment and I'm here on a mission of discovery," then you cannot fail. Experimentation removes the possibility of failure.

You can experiment with all sorts of things. You might try cooking something exotic. It's just an experiment. Who cares if it doesn't turn out as planned? You can try shopping at a farmers' market. See if you enjoy the experience of talking to the people who are growing your food. See if the prices are different. Find out whether or not you enjoy the experience. Maybe you stock up on food for the week and you cook all of your own meals. It doesn't really matter; it's just an experiment.

III.

Experimentation helps to focus your attention on something new and allows you to safely go outside your comfort zone. You continue to do the same old things because you do not want to try and possibly fail at something new. You must be coerced into doing anything new through motivation. This is how all fad diets start. The only way they can get you to try a new diet is by making fantastic claims. If the claims are not incredible, you will not be motivated enough to leave your comfort zone and try something new. Your fear of failure is too great.

Let's talk about the fear of failure. Why are you so concerned with failing? What effect does failing actually have on your life? It actually has no more effect than the label you place on it. Failure is simply a name given to an action that does not yield the results expected. But is that really bad? Of course not. It just seems bad from your limited perspective. If you look back at anything you've tried and failed at, you can see that the experience led you to something else. The experience was the prize of the activity and the label of failure is just a description that was created based on an unexpected result.

There is no such thing as failure. To redefine the word failure, you might call it an "unexpected outcome for which I am using a limited perspective to judge the results." From the higher perspective, you cannot fail, because all experience further defines your desires and thus clarifies and focuses your attention to what is wanted. The universe sees the intensity of your focus and you engage universal powers to bring you what you want, as long as you allow it.

Failure causes focus. The universe sees your focus and brings you the manifestation of your desire, as long as you allow it. When you believe that you have failed at something, you are resisting the experience as well as the clarification the result has caused within you. The failure is beneficial, not detrimental. You need not fear failure; you should indeed embrace it.

However, you label failure as wrong and judge yourself unfavorably, and this brings up negative emotion. When you fail, you believe that either you or the circumstances surrounding the experience is bad or wrong. This is a view that is not aligned with how your inner self sees the same situation. You feel like you failed and that is a bad thing, while your inner self sees your failure as a good thing. You look at things from the limited perspective and so to you it appears as if the failure is unwanted. Your inner self looks at everything from the higher perspective and understands exactly how everything is working out and why the experience of failure is so beneficial.

You have created a persona. This persona is your idea about who you are. However, it is false. It is a mere fragment of who you really are. It is just a glimpse of the real you. Who you really are is a limitless being of pure positive love and acceptance, free from fear. Who you are being, represented by your persona (or your idea of self), is fearful and limited. Your ego protects your persona just as the survival instinct protects your life. Your ego is under the false belief that the persona must be kept intact. However, if you are to become the version of you who is ready for your desires to manifest, you must change and your persona must change as well.

If you are to fail and you judge failure as a bad thing, then your persona runs the risk of being damaged by failure. Your ego will not allow this. Your ego is there to protect the persona. Your ego will keep you from doing anything where you might fail just so it can maintain the status of the persona. Your ego is the reason you don't want to leave your comfort zone.

If you are to try something new, it had better work. You do not want to risk failure, because you believe failure is bad. Your ego brings up many fears warning you of the danger of trying something new. You believe that failure is a bad thing and your ego is simply protecting you from what you think is bad. If you did not believe that failure was bad, your ego would not need to protect you from failure. It is your limiting beliefs that inspire your ego to keep bringing up all these irrational, fearful thoughts.

The diet industry understands this mechanism. They know that you are likely not to try anything new because you fear failure. In order to motivate you to try something new, they must entice you with detailed and numerous stories of success. They must demonstrate that the possibility of failure is extremely low. The only way to get you to do something is to remove the idea that failure is a possibility. In doing so, they create conditions that all but ensure failure.

It's a paradox. They make claims that they cannot possibly live up to so that you believe you cannot fail and then you try the diet because the possibility for failure appears to be nonexistent. Since the results cannot be achieved, you end up failing and your limiting beliefs about failure (and dieting and your ability to create a lean body) are intensified.

The only way to get the results you desire is to become a vibrational match to those results. That's it. It can happen instantly or it can take a lifetime. It's really up to you. If you remain safe in your comfort zone because you fear the feelings associated with failure, then you cannot become a vibrational match to what you want. However, if you can reduce the intensity of your idea about failure in general, you will allow yourself to come out of your comfort prison and you will try something new. The new thing will challenge your beliefs. If you resist the challenge, you won't alter your beliefs and therefore your vibration will not change. If you allow the new thing to challenge your beliefs and you come out the other side thinking about things in a new way, then you've allowed the change to take place and you're ready for the next step.

Experimentation is a device that will help you alter your beliefs about failure.

IV.

Bring yourself out of your comfort prison and try new things. Do not fear failure. Do not fear the alteration of your persona. Do not fear change. You must change your approach to life, your perception of reality, and who you are being in order to receive anything you desire. If you want something and it does not exist in your life now, you will literally have to change in order for it to enter your reality. You change to match the thing you want and the thing you want will come to you. This is the Law of Attraction.

You are resistant to what you want. Why is this so? Wouldn't it make sense to simply allow everything you want to come to you? Why in the world would you resist the thing you want so much? It's simply because you do not realize you're resisting it. If you knew what resistance really is, you could easily stop doing those things and instead start allowing. Allowing is the opposite of resisting. Experimentation lets you know whether you are actually allowing the change to take place or whether you're resisting it.

You want a lean body. You do not have a lean body now. In order to receive what you want, you must become a vibrational match to the version of you who has a lean body. How is that version different from the current version? The lean version of you obviously has a different set of beliefs, feelings, thoughts, attitudes, moods, and a different approach to life than the not-so-lean version that exists right now. How do you move from here to there? What are you to do?

Simply put, you must start to change your set of beliefs, feelings, thoughts, attitudes, moods, and your approach to life. The beliefs you hold onto, which keep your vibration at its present frequency, are contrary to those that you would have if you were the leaner version of yourself. There are a million different beliefs, attitudes, feelings, and thoughts that keep you from all that you want, including a lean body. You can work on those and you will gradually create a new reality. But before any of that can happen, you must change one thing first. You must radically change your approach to life from one who resists change to one who allows change.

There are only two approaches to life. The first approach is the one you were taught at a very early age. It is the one where you must change anything you think is bad or wrong. It's the approach where you fight against the conditions you don't like. Where you eradicate anything that seems unpleasant. Where you avoid any condition or situation where there might be a possibility of experiencing negative emotion. Where you hide your feelings and soothe yourself by reacting to the outside conditions. Where you believe that you are a victim of fate and that you really have no control over your life. Where you take no responsibility for the things that appear in your reality.

The radically new approach to life is one of allowing. You understand that you create your own reality and you take responsibility for and pride in your own creation. You understand that you are worthy and unique. You realize that there are no accidents, fate, or coincidences. You understand that everything is right and anything judged as wrong is done so only from a limited perspective. You know that from the higher perspective, everything is right the way it is. You understand that everything is always working out for you. This isn't just a comforting phrase; it is the design of physical reality and can be no other way.

The first approach to life is resistant and the second approach is allowing. To believe that something is wrong (including your present state of being) is a limiting belief. It is resistant in nature. It is false. It is based in fear. To believe that everything is right (including your present state of being) is nonresistant in nature. It is true. It is based in love. It is the basis of the universe. It is how the system was designed.

Resistance keeps you from changing into the version of you that is a match to your desire.

When you feel negative emotion, you are resisting. You are looking at the situation in a way that causes you to resist change. Now, if you can understand that the event that causes you to feel bad is actually there to help you see things from another perspective, you can ease your resistance and identify the fear that is at the root of your limiting belief about the subject at hand. As you know by now, that belief (along with others like it) is what is holding you apart from your desire.

The idea here is that you don't really know which beliefs are keeping you from which desires. You have many desires and many limiting beliefs. Some of the beliefs are so strong that you will have tremendous difficulty seeing them as limiting. Your key is to understand that anytime you feel negative emotion, you are uncovering a limiting belief. Even if you believe it to be a fact that is inscrutable, it is false if it's based on an irrational fear.

Experiment with your belief system. Allow your beliefs to be challenged. Experiment with your mood. Allow your mood to be elevated. Experiment with your feelings. Think about how you feel and see if you can't make yourself feel better. Experiment with your ability to manifest things. See if you notice when the time is aligned on a digital clock. Take notice that when you elevate your mood you encounter friendly people. Notice that when you set your intentions, everything just falls into place.

V.

Have you ever experimented with food? Do you know which foods are of value to your body? Do you understand that the foods you eat must be compatible with your specific and unique body so that the energy can be distributed throughout the system that is your body? Do you believe that every body is the same and therefore all foods are good (or bad) for all bodies? Your body is unique and you are a positive match to certain foods and not others. Experimentation will help identify the foods that are most easily absorbed by your unique body.

You are not your body; you simply are the captain of the "Earth Suit" that is your body. Your body is an organization of cells. Each one is seeking and finding balance and well-being. You have influence over your body through your thoughts. You think a thought and the body responds. You can think the thought to wave your hand and the body responds to your command. You can think a thought of despair and your body responds. You do not control most of the functions of the body. The body is intelligent and understands what it needs to do to survive. Without the collection of cells that make up the community that is your body, you could not experience physical reality.

Your body takes much of its form and shape based on thoughts you think now and the intentions you had prior to your arrival on Earth. You chose your specific body and its collection of attributes, talents, and even its apparent flaws. You chose the good aspects and even those things you consider to be wrong. You chose it all.

If you chose a body that was tall, this was done for a reason. You chose the sex and color of the skin for a reason. You chose the eye and hair color. You chose the talents or the lack of talent, the features of the face, the shape of the nose, the teeth, the size of the feet. If you were born without one or more physical senses, you chose that too. You chose it all because you knew that the specifics of your body would cause certain desires to unfold that would set you on a trajectory toward that which you came here to explore.

Your body is perfect as it is. Anything you deem as bad or wrong about your body is done so because you do not realize that you crafted it to be this way so that you could explore the world from the perspective of someone who inhabits your specific body. Having said that, there is a version of your body that is fully aligned with who you really are. This is the version of your body that would exist in its natural state, free from the influence of your limiting beliefs about it.

Your body reacts to your thoughts. If your thoughts are positive and pure, then your body allows well-being and balance is achieved. In this state, the size, shape, and health of the body is the perfect representation of what you intended prior to coming to this reality. Not all people choose a supermodel's body. In fact, very few do. The life experience created by a body like that is a specific one and would not allow you to explore reality as you intended (unless you are or were a supermodel). You chose the body you have for a very intentional reason.

Along the way your resistant thoughts influenced your body away from its natural state of health, well-being, and vitality. If you feel a lack of energy, it's due to your resistant thoughts and limiting beliefs. If you have gained weight, it's due to the thoughts you consistently think. If you have a chronic physical ailment, it's because you have a chronic pattern of resistant thought. If your body is addicted to something, it has only to do with your addictive habit of thought. Your body (and your reality) match how and what you are thinking. Change your body by changing the way you think.

You have a certain belief about food that is based mostly on bad advice. You have been told that every body is similar and that what is good for one is good (or bad) for all. This is not true. The fundamental truth is that you are unique and so is everyone else. This is quite obvious. So then, if you are unique, wouldn't it make sense that what's good for you may not be good for others and vice versa? What works for you is for you and what works for others is for them.

You have a unique vibration. When your vibration interacts with something, that interaction is unique because your vibration is unique. Imagine you are a unique color. When you mix the color that is you with the color orange, a new and equally unique color will be created. This is how it is with everything. When you eat a banana, the energy created by the combination of you and the banana is unique. It is not good or bad; it is simply unique. This energy may be readily accepted by your body or not. It does not depend on how others react to bananas; it has to do with how you respond. If the energy that is created is good for your body, you will feel it. If it is not, you will feel that too, as long as you are paying attention.

Your beliefs play a role in all of this. Your body might not easily absorb the energy created when you eat a banana. However, you believe that bananas are good in general and so you simply accept that the banana is good for you. It may very well be, but you cannot know until you experiment.

You may respond favorably to alcohol or you may not. How does alcohol make you feel? Every different type of alcohol has a unique vibration.

Experimentation

You might not react well to any of it no matter the dose. You might react very well to all of it. There might be some forms of alcohol that you cannot tolerate, but others that are more tolerable. Without experimentation, you cannot know.

You do not eat the same food as your dog or cat. You can easily see that they are very different than you. However, just as your dog is different, so is your neighbor, your friend, and your parent. What works for them has nothing to do with what works for you. You are unique. Treat everything you eat as a unique combination of your vibration and its vibration. Determine for yourself what works and what doesn't. Do not blindly accept that some foods are good and others are bad. If your body is not currently at its natural shape, it's because your belief about the foods you are eating must be challenged.

The question is not which foods are good and which are bad. Rather, the question is which foods are readily accepted by your unique body and which are not. Which foods give you energy and vitality and which foods do not? Since you are not really paying attention to the energetic exchange that is taking place while you eat, you cannot really know which foods work for you. That is why we ask you to experiment.

You do not know if your body can readily absorb the energy in a slice of bread. Maybe it can and maybe it can't. You have certain beliefs about bread. You might think that bread is good for everyone and therefore it's good for you. Certainly, this is a beneficial belief and to the extent to which you believe this statement to be true, it's true for you. However, you have been receiving some alternative information and this may have impacted the strength of your belief. You may think that gluten is bad and therefore bread is bad for you. But until you experiment, you cannot know. Knowing is strong belief. Convince yourself whether something is good or bad for you through personal experience and make your dietary decisions from that unique standpoint.

To test whether a food item is good for you, you must pay attention to what you are eating. If you were to eat a sandwich, would you know if your body accepted the energy exchange of the bread? No, because the sandwich is a combination of many different ingredients. To test if the bread component of the sandwich is accepted by your body, you must eat a slice of bread by itself. Now, here's the important part; the slice of bread you choose also contains many different ingredients because it has been processed. In order to know if that composition of ingredients called bread is good for you, you have to know that it is made the same way every time. Whole wheat bread from one company is different than whole wheat bread from another because the ingredients and the recipe are slightly different. However, if you were to make bread yourself using the same recipe and ingredients over and over, you could test how your body reacts to that bread and thus you would know if it was or was not easily accepted by your body.

It is easier to understand if a single, unprocessed food item is easily absorbed by your body. Eat an apple. How do you feel? How do you feel before you take the first bite? How do you feel while you're eating it? How does it taste? How does it feel in your mouth? How does it feel in your throat? How does it feel five minutes after you've eaten it? How do you feel one hour later? Do you believe apples are good for you? Notice your energy level after eating it. Now then, after all this experimentation and analysis, how do you feel about apples?

Apples of all varieties have generally similar vibrational qualities. Apples are apples and oranges are oranges and their frequencies are consistent enough that you can test how your vibration interacts with the vibration of the apple or orange. It is important to note how you feel after eating the fruit by itself. Eat an apple one day and then eat an orange the next day. Does one feel better than the other? Do you have more energy from one over the other? How do you feel an hour after eating it? These are questions you may have never asked before. The answers might surprise you.

When eating something raw, like an apple or any piece of fruit, you can understand the interaction between your vibration and its vibration and you can easily determine if your body accepts the energy of the fruit or not. However, when foods are cooked, the vibration is altered. The vibration of a cooked apple is very different than the vibration of a raw apple. The vibration of something is different depending on its state. The vibration of ice is different than steam. This is an obvious example. The vibration of canned tuna is different than fresh tuna.

Your vibration is unique, so it does not matter what others think or believe. What is good for you is due to a unique combination of your vibration and the vibration of whatever food you eat. You are unique and so that interaction is always unique. If you feel good after eating or drinking something, if you have energy and vitality, then you can know that the food works with your body in a way that is beneficial. If you feel bad, sluggish, constipated, bloated, gassy, etc., then you know that the food is not being easily absorbed into your body.

If you have a condition that is a side effect caused by eating certain foods, then you know that your body is not vibrationally compatible with those foods. If you have indigestion, heartburn, acid reflux, or anything else, you must be aware that the energy exchange is not going smoothly. There is some resistance on the part of your body. It is a message telling you that it's time to think about what you are putting into your body.

Typically, you are more concerned with the taste of the food or the way it makes you feel while you're eating it rather than the energy it will bring. If the food can distract you from the way you are feeling for just a bit, then that is what drives your decisions. The food may indeed be readily accepted by your body or it may not be. There's really no way to tell unless you do some experimentation.

Start with a list of foods you believe are good for you and as a snack each day, try one food and see how you feel. You want to make sure that you eat the food by itself. If you are testing whether or not a potato is good for you, you must cook it and eat it without salt, butter, or anything else. Just eat some of the plain, cooked potato and notice how you feel five minutes after you've eaten it. Then pay attention to how you feel an hour after. Did the potato taste good just by itself? Did you experience energy that lasts? Did you feel your mood shift? Were you able to think clearly? Did you feel an itchy sensation in your throat or anywhere else? If the item is vibrationally accepted by your body and the exchange of energy is completed with ease, then you will feel good. If not, you will receive information and feedback that will be noticeable if you are paying attention.

After you have confirmed that your body readily accepts the energy of the food, you can now experiment to see if it works in combination with something else. This time you will eat the potato with a sprinkle of salt. Now how do you feel? It will taste better because your taste buds are conditioned to eating a lot of salt. But think about how you feel five minutes and an hour after. Did you receive the same feeling of energy and vitality, or was there a difference? Did you notice any side effects? Was your mood altered in any way. Did you feel hungry soon after eating the potato or did you remain satisfied longer? There are no right or wrong answers. Simply pay attention to how you feel and you will learn by experimentation what your body likes and what it doesn't.

VI.

Experimentation is a device you can use to test the strength of your beliefs. Right now you have a set of beliefs about food that plays a critical role in which foods you will and will not eat. Your body is a representation of your beliefs about the foods you eat. You may be eating or avoiding foods based on your beliefs. Your body's current state is a result of your current set of beliefs. Alter those beliefs and the shape and condition of your body will change.

If you truly believed that eating fast food was good for your specific and unique body while simultaneously understanding that other people do not react well to fast foods, you could be perfectly lean and healthy eating fast foods for the rest of your life. It has to do with the beliefs about the foods you eat rather than the actual foods themselves. If you truly believe that something is good for you, then your body will adjust to accept that food and will readily and easily convert it to the energy it needs.

Your body will drive you to choose the foods it wants through the mechanism of urges and cravings. If you are in a positive emotional state of being and you are completely happy with the body you have, you will be inspired to consume those foods the body wants through cravings and other inspiration. However, if you are in a low emotional state of being and you are unhappy with the present state of your body, you will receive urges that are designed to distract you from how you are feeling. The urges will be for foods (or drinks, drugs, actions, etc.) that will temporarily cause you to feel better. However, they are only temporary and are counterproductive. They will not move you in the direction of that which you desire.

If you like the shape and condition of your body, your body will inspire you to choose the foods that it wants to keep you feeling and looking good. As long as you believe that what you are eating is aligned with how you feel about yourself, then everything you choose will work to maintain or even improve your present state. However, if you have doubts or fears about what you are eating, your body will have to work around those fears and side step your limiting beliefs.

You might believe that kale is good for you and so you eat kale because you think it will make you healthy. This is an example of a very beneficial belief. When your body wants the beneficial nutrients found in kale, it will inspire you to make a dish (or order one) that includes kale. Conversely, you might think that white potatoes are bad for you. You love the taste of a potato, yet you have a limiting belief that they are not good for you because somewhere along the line you read or heard something negative about potatoes. Now, if your body wants something beneficial that is found in potatoes, it must find a different food that conforms to your beliefs.

When you are presented with a potato in a meal at a friend's house, you feel conflicted. Your belief about the potato and your belief about being a good guest are now at odds with one another. So you eat the potato and due to your limiting belief, your body has a more difficult time accepting the potato. It has to do with your set of beliefs, not the food itself.

You have infinite beliefs about the foods that are available to you. Some are highly beneficial and some are quite limiting and most fall somewhere in between. Until you experiment with your personal and unique body and the foods you love, you cannot know which foods are right for you. Forget everything you've been taught. Forget everything you've heard. There is no right or wrong food for everyone. Everyone is different. All you need to know is what is good for you and you can leave the rest alone.

Experimentation will alter your beliefs in a way that will be for your benefit. Create a food journal. In this journal write a list of foods that you believe are good for you. Now, take one food from that list and complete an experiment every day. Within a month you will know how you feel about most of the foods you believe are good for you. Take notes in your journal and rate each one on a scale of one to ten. If your body does not feel good after eating it, then that food item ranks as a one. If your body accepts it easily and you feel good while eating it and afterwards, then that food item ranks as a ten.

You will find that some foods you believed were good might not be easily accepted by your body. It's not that you were wrong or that the food itself is bad, it's just that there might be a better alternative. You do not have to abandon the food completely; simply know that it doesn't interact with your body as well as some other foods do. You can eat it occasionally if you are inclined to, but maybe not as often as before.

Next you will list all the foods you love to eat but you believe are bad for you. Again, if you think that a hamburger is bad for you, you must experiment with each component by itself. One day you will eat the cooked patty by itself and note how you feel before, during, and especially after you've consumed it. Then you eat the bun on the following day. Then you try the ketchup, then the pickle, then the tomato, and so on until you've sampled and experimented with each ingredient. It may be that your body felt good with every item except the tomato. Thus, your body readily accepts hamburgers as long as there is no tomato. That might be quite a belief-altering experiment and could positively impact the rest of your life.

If you believe that a certain food is good, it is good for you. If you believe it is bad, then it is bad for you. However, you have never really experimented with most of the foods you eat on a regular basis. You simply assume that some things are good and others are bad. Until you experiment with your own body, we will submit to you that your limiting beliefs about those foods are false. Experiment to find out the truth about food for yourself and as a result, the beliefs that were created through experimentation will be highly beneficial.

Chapter Thirteen

How You Feel Is The Only Thing That Matters

If you think about it, the only thing you are ever doing while alive on this planet is feeling something. If you stop and think about how you feel right now as you are reading this book, how would you describe it? Are you feeling good? Are you anxious or worried? Are you cozy and secure? Do you feel loved and appreciated? Do you feel hungry or satiated? Are you tired? Are you interested? Are you enjoying this book?

How you feel is the only thing that really matters, because this is a feeling reality and all you are ever doing is feeling something. No matter where you are, who you're with, or what you are physically doing, all you are doing is feeling. If you can create the intention and desire to feel good, then due to the Law of Attraction, you will attract more good-feeling experiences and things. Your only work is to work on feeling as good as you can as often as you can.

Your senses bring you feedback about the physical world, but they don't cause how you feel. You determine how you feel by your own interpretation of the feedback you are receiving. If you feel good, you are interpreting your reality from a perspective that allows you to feel good. If you feel bad, you are looking at the outside conditions from a limited perspective that causes you to feel bad. It's your perspective, so it's always your choice.

If you were sitting on a hill in a meadow surrounded by nature and removed from any fear, you would feel good. Your natural state of being, free from the pressures and stress of your society, is one of well-being. Your natural set point is one that feels really good. You were designed to feel good. It is your birthright to feel good. Feeling good is an important part of living in physical reality. Everything you want in life is for one reason only: you think that the having of what you want will cause you to feel good.

You risk feeling bad so you can feel good. You might bet on a horse race in the hope of winning. If you win, you know you'll feel good. If you lose, you might feel worse than you did before you made the bet. You might ask someone for a date. You think that if the person says yes, you will feel better than you do now. If they say no, you might feel worse. It's a gamble, but the gamble to feel good is often worth the risk.

You might not bet on a horse race because if you lost, you would feel foolish and this is not worth the risk. You might not ask the person for a date because their rejection would feel worse to you than the excitement you might receive if they were to say yes. Everything is a trade-off depending on how you think you will feel as a result of the action. Many people experience wonderful and exciting things because to them the feelings associated with failure are not so acute. If they are rejected, they find a perspective that allows them to feel better quickly. If they fail, they look at the beneficial aspects of the failure and they move on. They are not afraid of the risk and so they do not let fear prevent them from trying something that has the potential to bring great joy.

Other people remain in their comfort zone paralyzed in fear because the thought of rejection, loss, or failure is so scary it prevents them from doing anything. They are happy staying where they are because the risk of feeling worse is too great.

In order to receive that which you want out of this life, you must learn how to deal with negative emotion. The only way you can feel bad in any situation is by choosing a perspective that is not in alignment with your inner self. As long as you can find the perspective that aligns with the way your inner self sees the situation, you will reduce the intensity and the duration of negative emotion.

II.

Imagine that from this day forward you decided that the most important thing is how you felt in every moment of the day. If you were determined to feel good, how would that look? What would you do? If it was your priority in life to simply feel good, you would start with how you deal with your emotions. The only thing that ever causes you not to feel good is negative emotion. Without negative emotion, you would naturally feel good. However, you do not want to rid yourself of bad-feeling emotions because that is half of your guidance system. You simply want to manage your response to negative emotion.

If you can realize that negative emotion causes you to feel bad, and your goal is to feel good, then all you have to do is create a system that shortens the duration of the negative emotion and reduces the intensity of it. Negative emotion arises when you feel fear. The fear is brought on as a response system when the structure of your persona is under attack. Since the persona is false, the fear is also false. If you can realize that negative emotion is always a gift because it allows you to see how your persona (and the limiting beliefs that support the persona) is trying to defend an indefensible aspect of the persona, you can use this to strip away the fear and alter your perception of who you are.

In other words, you have created this persona that is a limited idea of who you are. In order to receive that which you want, you must remove some of the limiting qualities of the persona. The ego defends the persona and tries to keep it intact. The ego believes that you have survived this long with this persona, so it does not want you to change. That's perfectly understandable, but it is limiting. If you want something and you don't have it in your life now, your persona must be changed.

If you could get to the point where you embraced those occasions where you felt negative emotion, and you could know that this is your opportunity to change, then negative emotion would not feel so bad. You would have a new perspective. You would see that the negative emotion is just there to guide you. It feels bad, but that's okay and it won't feel bad for long because you are quick to adopt a higher perspective that allows you to feel relief and return to feeling good.

Let's say that someone you love said something that hurt your feelings. In the past you would have felt angry or sad, blamed them for not being considerate, and held onto some resentment for a period of time. The initial comment felt bad, but your limited perspective caused the bad feeling to last for hours, days, or even longer. You might still remember an occasion when someone said something mean to you. You are still holding onto that (and many other hurtful comments) to this day. This is the feeling of resentment and it is always with you to some degree. This resentment causes you to consistently feel bad. If you can realize what you're doing, you can forgive the people who said those things. If you can realize that it was something you needed to hear so that you could alter your own limiting beliefs about yourself, you could then see that these hurtful comments were created to help you change your persona.

Make a pact with yourself that from this point on you will no longer choose the limited perspective when it comes to what people say around you. If they say something to you that you do not like, it's because the universe inspired them to say it so that you could uncover a limiting belief about yourself. Some of these beliefs are buried deep within you. You will not agree with them initially. You will try to make them wrong for speaking those words. However, if they said it and you heard it, it is for your highest good. You can realize that there is something to those words. You hold a belief that corresponds to what they said about you. Think about it and realize it's just another limiting belief and then do the work to reduce the intensity of that belief.

To feel good you must know that bad-feeling emotions are very good things. If you keep resisting and fighting the messages contained in your emotions, you will feel bad for longer periods of time. Imagine if you could get to a place where when someone says something hurtful, you could embrace it with love. That is true power. There is nothing more powerful than that. If you could see it for what it really is, you would easily slip off the limiting aspects of your persona and allow it to continually shift and move and change so that you could become a vibrational match to everything you ever wanted. Anything less than that is simply resistance.

We will say it again: you are not a match to what you want and that is proven because what you want does not exist in your life. In order for you to receive it, you must become a match to it. The universe will work to mold your belief system by creating events, comments, situations, etc. that bring up fear for you. You feel fear and this is manifested as negative emotion. The fear is irrational and comes in defense of the persona. The ego protects the persona by resisting the event. It makes you think that what is happening or being said is wrong.

If what was happening was right, then that means that you are holding onto a belief that is limiting. The belief is about yourself. Somewhere down deep inside you believe it also, otherwise you wouldn't get upset if someone said it. Imagine that you believe yourself to be a nice person. On the surface, this seems like a beneficial belief and in many respects it is. However, if you also believed that you were not nice enough, not good enough, not worthy enough, and someone said you were not nice, you would feel fear because the person has attacked the cornerstone of your persona. Your ego defends it by making the person who said it and their words wrong. You fight back. In this reaction you are not nice and your ego must fight on even harder.

If you could just give up your attachment to this one meaningless aspect of yourself, you would strip away the limitation it causes. You do not need to be nice or prove that you're good. You are a being of pure positive love and acceptance. Being nice is the least of your qualities.

If someone said you were not nice, and you felt no negative emotion, then you would know that you hold no limiting beliefs about yourself in this area. That is the method by which you can determine whether you have a limiting belief. If someone called you a bad driver and you felt bad, it's because being a good driver is a false aspect of your persona and you are trying to hold onto it. You are a being of pure positive love and acceptance. It is not important to you if people think you're a good driver or not. You are much more than that and being a good driver does not define who you are in the least.

If someone were to call you a bad bullfighter or a bad ballerina, you would not care because you are not defined by that. You would feel no negative emotion. You would probably laugh. This is the test. If you feel any negative emotion, you are holding onto a limited aspect of your persona and you can release it.

Imagine you are a stay-at-home parent and you care for your two children while your mate works outside the house. If your mate comes home and notices something about the children and says something, how do you think you would feel? You might feel negative emotion if you believed that being a good parent was the cornerstone of who you really are. You might get defensive in order to protect the appearance of this aspect. You might fight back and call your mate a name. You might choose to attack his or her role as the provider. In turn, he or she becomes defensive and the argument escalates as each party attempts to protect their own persona.

However, if you are secure in knowing that all you are is a being of pure positive love and acceptance, you could never feel negative emotion when attacked because you have no limiting beliefs about yourself. If you are a stay-at-home parent and you believe this role defines you, then you have just limited yourself. While this is one loving aspect of who you really are, it is just a tiny piece. You are much more than this.

Managing your emotions means understanding why you feel bad in the first place. If you did not fear that you were not good enough, you could not feel negative emotion. If you were to tell a race car driver that he or she was a bad driver, they would laugh. They would not care what you say. They know they are a good driver. There is no doubt or fear.

If you feel negative emotion, then fear exists. You are not as confident as you think you are. There is doubt. Either gain more confidence or do not consider that aspect of your persona to be defining.

III.

You will always face fear, your ego will always try to protect your persona, and your guidance system will never stop working. You do not need to shy away from negative emotions; all you need to do is understand their role and what is really happening when you feel bad. Your natural set point is one of well-being. This is a state free from fear. Fear will pop up occasionally whenever you have a limiting belief that is preventing you from becoming a match to what you want. That's okay. That's part of the system. You very much want to be able to adjust your belief system (and your vibration) so that you can receive all that you want. You want to change because change means adjusting vibration in order to receive something wanted.

Feeling good is your natural state. If you can remember times in your childhood when you did not worry or have a care in the world, that was your natural state of being. Unfortunately, you were told that the world is scary, that you must struggle to be successful, that you must work hard, and that you must behave and conform if you want to have a good life. This was never true, but you adopted these limiting beliefs and so you started your life-long habit of worry. Worry is a negative feeling brought on by fear and it is not true.

When you worry about something, you are imagining a false reality. You are thinking about the negative potential that could happen. You are creating your own fear. Since you cannot know what will happen, you use your imagination to assume the best (hope) or the worst (worry). Your future unfolds based on your vibration, not what you think should or could happen.

Everything is happening to bring you what you desire. If you had no desires, then you would not need to change who you were being, because without desire, there is no need to change. You might worry about the future, but then that would be a desire for something. If you were truly at peace with everything, having no desire whatsoever, then you could feel no negative emotion.

Negative emotion means that you are looking at something from a perspective that is not aligned with the person you need to become in order to receive what you want. Positive emotion means that you are looking at the subject from a perspective that is perfectly aligned with the person you are becoming who will be a match to your desire. If you have negative emotion, it means you have a desire. The stronger the negative emotion, the stronger your desire. If you feel strong negative emotion, it means that the desire is also strong and your perspective is completely different from the perspective you would have if you were a match to your desire.

If your desire is not too strong, the negative emotion will be mild. If the negative emotion is mild, that means that your perspective is just slightly off and the intensity of your limiting belief is rather weak. It is easier to regain a proper perspective when the emotion is mild than it is when the emotion is strong. You can alter your perspective rather easily when the emotion is something like boredom, apathy, or even frustration. However, when the emotion is anger, despair, hatred, or rage, the perspective is very far off and the limiting belief is highly intense.

We suggest you start with the mild emotions. Try to see the situation from another perspective. Realize that what you are feeling is not aligned with the version of you who will be a vibrational match to some desire. Know that your perspective is off, but not far off. You just need a little nudge to get back on track. Start thinking about what it is you fear here. When something happens, think about why you care. What does it really mean? Are you making something up? Is it even about you? See if you can identify the limiting belief about your persona that needs to make the event wrong. When someone says something, why are you choosing to view it as an assault on your personality? Instead, realize that you feel fear because your ego is just trying to validate some meaningless aspect of the persona. It just doesn't matter.

Feeling good starts with having a flexible persona. If your idea of yourself is rigid, then your ego will constantly need to protect the persona. For instance, if you believe yourself to be intelligent, then you will react in fear whenever your intelligence comes into question. You will instantly feel bad and from that low-emotional state of being, you will sabotage yourself by doing or saying things as a reaction to how you are feeling. You will take action to defend your false persona. This action which is inspired from a low-vibrational state of being, will be counterproductive and will not bring you closer to becoming who you must become to receive what you desire.

If you believe yourself to be intelligent, that is a beneficial belief as long as it is not limiting. Can a belief be both beneficial and limiting at the same time? Certainly. If you believe yourself to be intelligent, that is a beneficial belief. But if you believe that your intelligence defines you, that is a limiting belief. The limitations of that belief become apparent when your intelligence is questioned. If you feel negative emotion, you have uncovered the limitations of an otherwise beneficial belief. You are intelligent, you have access to higher and broader nonphysical intelligence, but you need not be defined by your intelligence.

Who you really are is a limitless being of pure positive love and acceptance. Anything less than that is your self-created persona, which is limited. Your persona limits who you can become if it is too rigid. If you are holding on defensively to certain aspects of that persona, then your persona is rigid and change is difficult for you. If you are not attached to any specific aspect of your personality, if you allow yourself to be flexible in your assumptions of who you are, you can change more easily.

Your persona must change in order to receive whatever it is you want. If you want a lean body, your idea of self must change from who you are being to who you will become. If you define yourself with any label, you place limitations on your idea of self. If you believe that your parents were fat and so you must have a metabolism that does not release fat easily, you've simply placed your own limitation on yourself. If you believe that you have a certain genetic condition, you've just limited yourself. All labels are self-imposed limitations and they are all false, no matter how strongly you believe they are true. By believing they are true, you simply engage the Law of Attraction, which proves them to be true for you.

IV.

You create your own reality. You create your own limitations. You create your own success. You created the body you have now and you can choose to deliberately create the body you prefer. You cannot escape the body you have now, for escape is not the most empowering perspective. You must lean in and become a match to the body you prefer and that body will begin to take shape. You must work with the set of beliefs you now have. You can adjust your beliefs in time and in time your body will take the shape you prefer. There's no need to rush. Losing twenty pounds in one month is not necessarily helpful. It may be helpful to the marketer of the diet, but it's not a vibrationally effective thing to do.

Typically, your vibration changes in subtle ways and so your life seems to be quite stable. You did not gain twenty pounds in one month; it was a gradual thing. You allowed your definition of who you are in your body to gradually change and now you are faced with a reality you do not prefer. So why would you think that shifting your vibration dramatically so that you could lose all the weight in such a short period of time would be effective? It would not. The change in vibration would not likely hold. You would revert back to your old vibration and your weight would return.

If you are inspired by something, you alter your belief and your reality is similarly altered. Your beliefs are changed. But in order for your beliefs to really change, you must be given evidence. Without evidence, you will go back to your old habit of belief and your world will change to reflect those old beliefs. If you are inspired to lose weight by a diet and you try it, your world temporarily changes because you are able to suspend belief for a little while, but then you find evidence that proves the diet is not working and you return to thinking the same old thoughts and so your body must also return to it's former state.

If you could alter your belief system permanently, your reality would shift permanently. This is the basis of this entire book. It is not your eating habits that you must change. It is not the amount of exercise that you must endure. It is not about your age, metabolism, genetics, or any of that. The only way to change your body (and your life in general) is by permanently changing your set of beliefs. In order to do that we suggest you radically change your entire approach to life.

If you can understand that it is your perception of reality that affects your health, your weight, your relationships, your wealth, and everything else, you can form a more empowering perception by looking at life in a new way. When you understand that everything happens for your benefit, you can allow the lingering effects of negative emotion to fade away. When you can understand that how you feel is equal to what you receive, then you can start feeling good today and start receiving all that you want. As soon as you can get our premise that nothing you want is achieved but that everything you want is received, you can switch your approach to life from one of trying and efforting, to one of feeling and allowing.

We are going to help you radically change your belief system so that you see your life from a much higher and broader perspective. We are going to convince you that you are indeed worthy and unique. We are going to alter your perception of yourself and the world around you. We are going to show you that a life of ease is far more effective than a life of struggle. We are going to work together in a coordinated fashion to change your mind about who you really are. The side effect of all this will be the body you want, the health you want, the abundance you want, and the relationships you want. You are a limitless being of pure positive love and acceptance and we are going to introduce you to who you really are.

Chapter Fourteen

Who You Really Are

You are an eternal, spiritual being who has chosen to come to Earth and explore physical reality in your own unique way. You are a worthy being, as worthy as any who have ever lived. You are unique to all the universe. Who you really are is a limitless being of pure positive love and acceptance. This is true of you and of everyone you know. However, you are experiencing life from a slightly more limited perspective.

If you knew the magnificence that is you, you could literally be, do, and have anything you wanted. If you understood fully that you create your own reality, you would utilize the knowledge of the powers of the universe, which you have access to now, to create whatever feeling you desire in the moment. You would hold how you feel as the most important aspect of physical reality and you would strive to feel good.

You would understand how your emotional guidance system works and you would know that as you birth a desire, you will be led along a path toward the manifestation of the desire. Along the path you would encounter manifestation events designed to help shape your belief system so that you could become a vibrational match to all that you want. When feeling any negative emotion, you would know that this is simply an indication that a limiting belief exists and you would analyze the fear at the base of it and prove to yourself that the fear was false. Your limiting belief would be lowered in intensity and your perspective would be raised, along with your vibration.

If you were to live in physical reality completely aware of who you really are, you would view nothing as wrong. You would find a perspective that would allow you to see things as right. You might not personally prefer certain things, but you would remove your attention from those things, knowing that they could be right for others. You would focus your attention on what you prefer and leave the rest alone. You would not fight against anything or make anyone wrong, including yourself. You would not judge another or yourself. As a being of pure positive love and acceptance, you would love and accept others and yourself as you are. In fact, you would consider everything as it is in the moment as perfect.

There is a reason you would love and accept everything in the moment as perfect. That's because it is perfect. If you cannot change anything in the moment (because in the moment it cannot be changed), then you must call it perfect. What is, is and that is perfection. It might be improved in time, but in the moment it is fixed, it cannot be changed, and it is perfect.

Living as who you really are would be living as an allower would live. You would not force things or struggle to push your way through; you would allow everything you want to come to you. You would become a receiver and not a doer. You know that this universe is set up to provide you with all that you want and that the only way something does not come to you is if you resist it. You know that change is not only good, but necessary and inevitable. You are constantly changing. There is no need to resist change. Change allows you to receive that which you want.

Living as the fullest version of who you really are in physical reality means you obey the rules of physical reality. You are aware of your fears. You know the difference between a rational fear and an irrational fear. You do not pet lions or jump off cliffs because your fear warns you that these activities could prematurely end your time in physical reality. However, you know that irrational fear is limiting and that you are a limitless being. You reduce the intensity of the feeling of fear by finding evidence that proves it is false. You see how it can be limiting and you shrug it off and move through the fear. The feeling you receive as a result is exhilaration.

This is the radically new approach to life we wish for you to embrace. This approach to life resonates with who you really are. It works within the laws of the universe and the mechanism of physical reality. It is a different way to look at life, but we promise you, it is so much more effective than your old approach. Just seeing the possibility of this new approach to life will cause a shift in your vibration.

II.

Start here:

Nothing is wrong. Everything is right. If you can live by this one statement, your life will get easier. A life of ease allows all that you want to come. Create ease in your life by starting to see how everything could be right. When your mate does something you do not like, instead of making them wrong, see how they could be right. You can't change anyone, even if you think you can. You are simply causing them to temporarily modify their behavior. When you ask them to be someone they are not, you are trying to change the conditions outside of you and this creates conflict and stress. Instead, change yourself.

Everything happens for you. If your mate does something you do not like, they did it specifically for you. That's how it is right. They are challenging your belief system. They are letting you peek into a limiting belief that is based in some irrational fear. Look at the fear rather than asking them not to do things that cause you to feel fear.

Do you understand what we are talking about here? If you ask them to behave in a way that does not cause you fear, you are just hanging onto a limiting belief. Your life is limited by this belief. You cannot get what you want as long as you hang onto this belief. You must release the limiting belief in order to vibrationally change so that what you want can come to you. By judging their behavior as bad or wrong and asking them to change instead of you, you do nothing to remove your own limitations. You are looking outside yourself and trying to change the outer conditions rather than taking a look inside and seeing how you could change instead.

Everything is right. If it is happening, it is happening for you no matter what it is. If you are aware of it, then it is for you. If you are not aware of it, then it is not for you. That's how you can tell. If someone says something nice to you, then that is for your benefit and growth. It reinforces a beneficial belief. If someone says something rude to you, then that is for your benefit, because it allows you to take a look at a limiting belief you have about yourself. It is always, always for you.

Everything is right for someone, somewhere. If it is not something you prefer, that's okay. Just remove your attention from it. It is not your place to decide what is good or bad, right or wrong for anyone else. They all came here to explore reality in their own way and they are all expanding as a result. Just because you cannot see the benefit of a life they chose doesn't mean that it is not a valid way to explore physical reality.

From your perspective you cannot see how some things might be right and that's okay. There are a lot of things going on in this world. That is by design. There have never been more people on the planet. That is because there has never been such diversity and opportunities for exploration. More are coming now because frankly there's a whole lot more to explore. Never before in the history of the planet could one explore such great wealth and abundance as well as such great poverty. Never could one have the opportunity to rise out of poverty to great wealth. Life on Earth has never been better from the perspective of those who come here to explore physical reality. If you can't see it as right, at least do not judge it as wrong.

Everyone is right and so are you. You are not wrong either. You cannot be wrong. If you say or do something that you or others judge as wrong, you are simply looking at it from the limited perspective. From the higher perspective, everything is right. You cannot fail. You have never failed. Everything you have ever done has been an act of expansion. Every result is one that causes expansion. You came here to expand and you are expanding. You are a success.

Where you are in life is not wrong either; it's perfect. You are at the right place and the right time. You are reading the right material for you. You are one of the few people on Earth to be interested in this information. That says something very important. The life you have led up to now has somehow allowed you to find this book. If you have been led to this book, then you are on your way to receiving much more than a lean and healthy body. You are on your way to an elevated vibration and your world will shift as a result. Have no regrets. Everything has worked out perfectly.

We ask that you understand fully the concept that you, yes you, are a limitless being of pure positive love and acceptance. You have the ability to love unconditionally. You can choose to accept all the actions and behaviors of those around you. This is unconditional love. You don't care about the conditions; you choose to love anyway. However, the most important love is self-love. Until you learn to accept yourself unconditionally, you will have great difficulty accepting others.

You are perfect as you are. You chose to explore life in the way you are exploring it. Everything is right. Everything has turned out perfectly. You are perfect as you are. We know this to be true. Any fault you see in yourself is not a fault at all. There is nothing wrong with you because there is no wrong anywhere in the universe. You are perfectly right in every single way. You are good.

This is the most important concept for you to know before moving forward. The lean body you desire, the abundance you desire, and the relationships you desire all start with love of self. It is good and right to love yourself. You are meant to love yourself above all others. To love yourself is to love others. The two ideas are unified. They are inseparable. You cannot truly love another more than your capacity to love yourself. If you love another truly, then you love yourself truly as well.

You could easily love yourself if you removed the conditions that appear to block that love. You have a perception of yourself that is false. It is a fallacy. It is not true. It is limited. Who you really are is a magnificent, limitless, eternal being. We are not kidding. When you make your transition to the nonphysical, you will come to understand that. You will look back on who you thought you were and you will wonder why you were so dazzled by the illusion that you were less than magnificent.

Others have led you to believe that you are less than perfect. That's just because they were trying to control the conditions and you happened to be one of those conditions they wanted to control. That's okay. It is quite a beneficial experience to peek behind the illusion and catch a glimpse of who you really are. It is fun to come from a low vibration and consciously move up the vibrational scale. It is exhilarating to move through fear to deliberately create the life you prefer. This is the opportunity that lies ahead of you now.

You are a limitless being of pure positive love and acceptance. To be loving is to be accepting. To accept others as they are means that you must first accept yourself as you are. You must accept yourself with all your qualities, some of which you judge as good and some you judge as bad. What are your good qualities? List them now. Take out a pen and paper and in your own hand write a list of your top twenty best qualities. Are you smart? Are you funny? Are you loyal? Are you giving? Are you talented in some area? Do you have good taste? Do you like animals? Can you see beauty? Are you creative?

Now you might also think about those qualities you do not appreciate. You might think of the things you want to fix. Are you overweight? Are you shy? Do you feel anxious? Do you worry? Do you feel fear? These, too, are positive qualities. Can you see how they are right? Can you see that your unique being is made up of a very unique set of attributes? But that is not who you are. You are not the sum of your good and bad qualities. You are much, much more than that. Your good qualities are good qualities and your bad qualities are simply limitations you place on yourself, but they are not true. You are all good. There is no bad. It's just a matter of your personal perception.

You believe that if you had a better mix of good and bad qualities, your life would be better. Your life is a representation of how you feel on the inside. It matters not who your parents were, where you were born, what you look like, or how intelligent you are. It is all a matter of how you feel about yourself and the world around you. Feel better about yourself and your world will shift to match how you feel. It all starts and ends with you. You are the only one who matters in your reality. Everyone and everything is simply a reflection of how you feel.

III.

This is why you must feel good. You must believe that there is a magnificent, eternal, limitless being of pure positive love and acceptance somewhere inside you. Unless you feel better about yourself, your life, your world, and everything else, you will simply continue to live a life of resistance. Everything you want is coming to you, but you are resisting much of it. You resist it by believing in your limited self, called your persona. The persona is false. It is simply a highly limited construct of who you think you are. Break down the false persona you think is so real and begin to see the magnificence that is really you.

When you believe yourself to be a pure positive being of love and acceptance, you will begin to think about yourself differently. When you strive to feel good above everything else, you will begin to see the world differently. When you accept the conditions as they are and begin to realize that everything is happening for you, you will be given clarity and you will be inspired to take action from a high emotional state of being. This is how you utilize the forces of the universe to deliberately create the lean body you desire, as well as everything else.

You are trapped in a body you don't like because you don't like it. It's as simple as that. Your focus is on what you do not like. We are not going to tell you what to do to lose weight. We are not going to give you a list of good and bad foods. We are not going to tell you what exercises to do. But we are going to give you one assignment: you must come to appreciate who you are and you must learn to accept the conditions that surround you (including your body) as perfect. Until you do, you will continue resisting and the weight will not come off.

However, once you start accepting yourself as perfect, you will start to feel better. The momentum will build. You will start to feel good. When you feel good, you will be inspired. The inspiration may be to cook your own dinner tonight. It may be to take a walk. It may be to buy some new clothes. It may be to call a friend. Whatever it is, if it feels exciting or interesting, it may just lead you down a new path.

Certainly, you will encounter irrational fear, but you will learn to deal with it and move past it. You will find evidence that it is false and you will go ahead with your inspired idea, knowing that it is leading you to the next step. You will proceed and when you feel negative emotion you will know that this is just an indication of a limiting belief and you will stop and think about it. You will analyze the fear and say to yourself, "This is not rational. This is not real. This fear is false. This limiting belief came from someone else. I know this belief is not needed and I allow it to fade away."

You will act when inspired and you will listen for inspiration. You will not do things that are not interesting or fun because unless it seems interesting, exciting, challenging, or fun, it is not inspired. If it is hard, painful, tedious etc., it is not inspired. Forget what you've learned about working hard. Nothing is achieved through hard work; it is achieved through inspired action. Sometimes you like to be inspired to do something and you make it harder than necessary because you believe that it takes a lot of work and effort to see results. This is not true. Make it easy and fun and you will achieve things effortlessly.

When you act out of love rather than fear, you allow the universe to do the work for you. Your limiting beliefs are limiting what the universe can bring. Start thinking in a limitless way. Start thinking bigger. Start imagining that nothing can go wrong, for that is entirely accurate. If something goes wrong, it's simply pointing out another limiting belief. Don't worry, move ahead and be captivated by what unfolds. It is all within your power when you view yourself as a limitless being of pure positive love and acceptance.

Chapter Fifteen

Free Your Mind and Your Body Will Follow

You gained weight through resistance to what is. You will lose the weight when you drop your resistance. It is that simple. Your weight is a physical reminder that you are not allowing life to flow. You are going against the flow. Now, if you look around you, you can see resistance in most everyone else as well. Their resistance is carried on their bodies. When the resistance causes weight gain, then the resistance is obvious. If it causes drug, alcohol, sex, or any other addiction, it is not so obvious. Your specific set of beliefs allow you to soothe yourself by eating while other people have beliefs that allow them to soothe themselves with other substances or activities. The one you chose happens to manifest itself as weight gain.

Your mind is constructed by a pattern of thought that you choose to think over and over and over again. You think the same thoughts in the same manner day in and day out in a never-ending, momentum-building, stubborn fashion. These patterns hold you in place and work to resist the natural movement and change you intended before your birth into this reality. When you begin to change your thinking, you begin to alter your own reality.

You are a resistant person. The proof of that is to be found in your physical body. If you are overweight, it may be that you are resisting the way your life is unfolding and to soothe yourself you eat in a manner that is not perfectly aligned with who you really are. If you lived a life free from stress, pressure, and resistance, your body would take its natural shape. But the stress is causing you to find a way to soothe yourself. Instead of looking inward to relieve your stress, you have made it a habit to reach for something outside yourself. However, you don't realize one important fundamental rule of all this: stress is always self-created.

There is no real thing that causes stress. Your finances cannot cause stress unless you look at them in a way that brings up fear. Your boss or customers cannot cause you to experience stress. You must look at them and feel fear in order to cause your own stress. Your weight cannot cause you stress. You look at your weight and you use it as the excuse for so many of your perceived problems and dissatisfactions, but it is not the problem. It is all in your mind.

Your habit of looking at life from a limited and fearful perspective is all that causes stress. It's just a habit of thought and nothing else. Those without stress do not gain weight or soothe themselves with outside stimulants. They are free of that habit. They live easily with a perspective that is aligned with who they are. They live without feeling irrational fear. These are the lucky ones. They have somehow managed to find a way to see the world from a higher perspective. They are natural-born allowers and they naturally live within the laws of the universe. They are the few. The rest of you live with some form of stress every day of your life. It is time to free yourself from this limited perspective and reduce the amount of irrational fear in your life. Once you do that, your body will return to its natural healthy and vibrant state of being.

All stress is created by thinking in terms of fear rather than love. When you believe you must do something or something bad will happen, that's fear. You cannot know what will happen, so you worry. The worry causes stress and inner conflict because it goes against the nature of your natural state of well-being. When you feel stress, you look for something to improve how you are feeling. You think this is an effective remedy from what you have learned about dealing with stress. The stress is mild and the cure seems easy enough. Just find something, anything, to distract you from how you are feeling. But whenever you look outside yourself to fill that feeling of dread, you are simply affixing a temporary patch. As soon as your mind returns from the distraction, you start to fret and worry all over again. The stress always returns.

If you had a million dollars in the bank, you believe that would ease your stress and to a certain extent and in a specific part of your life that might be true. If you are stressed out by the thought of paying your bills, then extra money would relieve that stress. However, this is an outside fix. It is the same as eating or drinking to relieve your feelings. It is not the permanent and effective way to fill the void. If the money allowed you to relieve your financial worries, it would do nothing to relieve your worthiness issues, your relationship doubts, or your low self-esteem, and in fact it might make your life even more stressful in other areas. There is no cure for an inner conflict in the outside world. It is an inside job.

If you have anxiety, the cure is inside you. If you feel empty, the cure is inside you. If you are stressed out, the relief is inside you. It is all there. All you have to do is figure it out. But once you do, you will discover the key to achieving anything you want in life. By solving the real issue, all the symptoms of stress disappear. All the extra weight will go away. All the anger and frustration that causes stress will vanish. All the problems in your life will be resolved once you understand how to meet the issue face to face in your inner world.

So, then, how do you specifically deal with your own stress? How do you learn to live life in a manner that allows you to remove the stress before it even starts? There is a process to all of this, but it requires you to think in new ways and to practice a new style of living. You must change how you've approached life. You must go in a totally new direction. You must do everything differently. You must believe that the old way is not effective for you. The old way is too hard. The old way is too much of a struggle. You must give in and realize that there is another way to live. We are asking you to forget everything you've ever learned about living a good life and we ask you to live a self-directed life.

A self-directed life is one where you place yourself first. We will tell you that physical reality is an illusion. It is a very convincing illusion. You believe you are one of several billion people living on this planet. You think you are an individual drop of water in a vast sea. You believe that you are not that important or special. But there is a secret. The secret is this: you are the center of your universe. You are worthy of everything you desire.

You are unique to all the world. You are really the only thing that matters in your universe. You are one with everything and are a unique expression of the Source. You must learn to place yourself above all else. You are in this adventure for your own personal growth and expansion. This is your life and your birthright is the opportunity to create your specific life in any way you choose. There is no one on Earth who is more important than you. You can have, be, and do anything you want. You are the supreme being. In order to understand how important you are, you must understand that you are the center of it all. Everything else revolves around you.

This is the design of physical reality. You have chosen to come to Earth at this time to explore reality in a new and fascinating way. You literally can do anything you like. There are no rules. Nothing is good or bad. You can judge for yourself what you want to do, what you enjoy, and what you prefer. It is all here laid out for you. There are no restrictions, none whatsoever. The only restrictions in this life are applied by you.

You are the only one who can limit what you get out of this life. Your beliefs about the way the world operates were adopted from those who had very little knowledge of how this all works. If you had been raised by a parent who knew this information, your set of beliefs would have been much more empowering. However, now you find yourself with a set of limiting beliefs. You can allow them to fade away. You do not have to be restricted by your own beliefs. You can adopt new, more empowering beliefs.

You came here to experience physical reality in a new and unique way. You have come many times before and this time you are looking at life from a new angle. In fact, no one else has ever experienced life as you are experiencing it now. It is unique in all of the universe. That's how you know that the universe revolves around you. Your experience is accepted by the universe as valid, worthy, and important. Without you and your experience, the universe would be less than it is.

In order for you to experience physical reality in a way that is unique to you, the system is set up to yield to your every desire. What would be the purpose of a physical reality where you could not grow as a result of a specific set of experiences? If you could not expand through the experiences you deem interesting and important, then physical reality would have no reason to exist. The main purpose of physical reality is to provide you with a means of personal expansion. In order to do that, it must be designed to provide infinite possibilities for exploration. In doing that, it must allow for you to receive that which you want. It is the basic design of the system.

Let this be your first belief that you hold above all else. You are a worthy being who came to experience physical reality in a unique way that would create the specific expansion you intended prior to coming here. You know that in order to experience physical reality in the way you intended, reality would have to bend itself to meet your desires. You now know that anything is not only possible, but if you want it, it must come to you. Everything you ask for is being delivered to you from the moment you decide it's something you want. That is the fundamental law of the universe.

The second belief that we want to impart to you is the fact that you can have, be, and do anything you want as long as you allow it. You can also birth a desire and choose not to allow it to come to you. This is part of the design of physical reality. If everything you wanted came to you the instant you thought of it, then anything you didn't want would also have to come to you as soon as you thought of it as well. You wanted to experience a reality where you allowed certain things to come but you also had a way to stop them from coming if you changed your mind. In this system you can choose any experience and then allow in those that you feel like experiencing.

You have gotten really good at the resisting part of the game. The resistance came mostly from not understanding your true worthiness. If you knew how magnificent you were, you would allow more of the good stuff in. But believe it or not, you are solely responsible for blocking all that you want from coming to you. It is all there waiting for you, but your limiting beliefs keep you from accepting it. That's okay, because you now have the opportunity to change your approach.

The reason you do not allow what you want to come to you is because you believe in right and wrong. For you personally, there are right ways to do things and there are wrong ways to do things. Some things are good and some things are bad. You judge this method for receiving what you want as good and this other method as bad. That's all fine; however, based on the beliefs you've adopted from others, it's limiting.

There is nothing wrong with living a limited life. That's how the vast majority of people operate. They are held prisoner by their own belief system. The tragedy is that most of your beliefs were adopted from others who had those same beliefs. You did not have the actual experience; you just listened to an old story and picked up the belief the same way you pick up a virus. Your body has defenses against a virus. We have shown you how to defend against a limiting belief. The question is whether you will do the work or not.

Everything you want is coming to you if you will just allow it. How do you allow what you want to come? You reduce your resistance. How do you reduce resistance? You believe that nothing is wrong or bad. If you believe something is wrong, you have just resisted it. If you think something is bad, you have just resisted it. Nothing is good or bad; it is all neutral. Your habit of judgment causes you to see good things as bad and right things as wrong. This is why you personally cannot get what you want. This is why you feel stress. This is why you feed your stress with food. This is why you gain weight. This is the cause of everything unwanted. This is the simple truth of physical reality.

II.

In an attractive reality such as this, non-resistance is the key to operating within the design of the system. All of the great successes in life come from working with the system rather than fighting against it. Some may enjoy the fight because it gives them a feeling of purpose, but the fight cannot give you what you really want. Nothing is wrong; it is always right. Things are perfect as they are now and improving with every new moment. Work within the system and you become an allower. Everything you personally want will flow to you while in the state of allowing.

You do not need to change anything. If you see something as wrong or bad, realize that it is simply your excuse for something that you feel is wrong in your life. If you believe that your bills are too high and you're not making enough money, that is simply your excuse for feeling bad. If you feel that no one loves you because your body does not look attractive, that is simply your excuse for feeling bad. There is nothing outside you that can cause you to feel bad; it is simply your habit of perspective. You see something and you blame your negative feeling on that. However, the thing you judge as bad is not bad, it's simply your excuse.

You can look at anything and feel good. You can use anything as your excuse to feel good. You can choose to enjoy life and feel good. You can also look at the things you lack and feel bad. You can look at the lives of others and by comparison you can feel bad. Feeling bad is easy. You've been doing it for a long time. However, unless you purposely choose to feel good, you will not change your life in a meaningful way. From now on you will do the work required to feel good.

Feeling bad has become a habit. You allow others to influence you to feel bad. You believe that how you feel is out of your control. We have come into your reality for one reason: to help you understand the importance of feeling good. Feel good and all you want will come to you. Choose to keep feeling bad and nothing changes. It just gets worse.

Your work is to find a way to feel good. It is not hard to feel good once you get started. It is your natural state of being. You simply have some momentum built up and this causes you to receive the same low-vibrational thoughts day in and day out. We are going to change that program. We are going to put in a new program. The new program is going to alter your perspective on life so that instead of focusing on the bad, you start focusing on the good. Instead of rushing to judgment, you are going to stop and think about the subject from another, more empowering perspective. Instead of complaining about something, you're going to find a way to praise it. The praising of things you don't like will help you receive things you do like. This is the new operating system.

Nothing is wrong, so there's no need to complain. There's no purpose in talking about what you do not like. This is your habit and it's contradictory. It goes against everything you want. The universe does not understand that you don't like something, but for some reason you enjoy talking about it. It doesn't make sense given the fundamental design of the system. Why would you put your attention on anything you don't like when your attention is the tool for bringing you more of whatever you are focused on? If you focus on something you do not like by talking about it, then all you are doing is asking the universe to bring you more of it. If you do not like it, if you think it's bad or wrong, don't talk about it; instead, find a way to see it as right or remove your attention from it.

If you can do this one thing, your life will radically improve. It will transform into something truly wonderful. Simply by refraining from complaining and instead working to see it in a positive light, your life will shift upwards so dramatically that you won't truly believe it. You might not believe that such a simple change in your approach to life could cause such a profound shift in your reality. But it is true. You see, by refusing to complain and then choosing to see the beauty in the ugly, you change your entire point of attraction. You raise your vibration from low to high with one simple change in your approach. You move from fighting against the system of reality to engaging the leverage of universal forces. You go from paddling upstream to floating downstream. It's as simple as that.

It might be a simple concept, but there's a lot of momentum and you have a habitual way of thinking and talking. It takes attention and practice. You will be the only one you know doing this work. You will be alone on an island. You will notice that you've attracted a group of people around you who approach life in the same old manner. They will continue to complain. They will continue to seek out the negatives. They will continue to soothe themselves with outside distractions and they will continue to urge you to do the same thing. They will not want to talk to someone who sees the world as positive and perfect. They won't want to talk about the same things you want to discuss.

You cannot change them, because that is fighting against what is and you have given that up. Your choice will be to stay with them and their approach to life or to understand that they might not change and you cannot change them. That's okay. Your work will be to stay out of it. If they choose to continue to complain, then that's their right. You cannot create in their reality; you can simply choose to see them as they are and love and accept them anyway. You don't need them to change in order for you to change. They will actually help you change because they will be a reminder of the old approach to life.

III.

You are a judge. You have been taught to judge. Accept that fact. You are very good at judging. You judge everything. Part of this habit of judgment stems from being physical. Your survival instinct causes you to constantly judge whether you are safe or not. You must inspect the food you eat because if you don't you might eat something that could kill you. You judge other drivers because if they make a sudden move, you could get into an accident. The ability to judge safe from unsafe is a valid aspect of your existence. It is right and good to judge.

However, when you judge something as wrong or bad when it is not a life or death matter, you place your perspective on one side of the subject. If you see it as right, then all is well. If you see it as bad or wrong, then you are resisting it. If it can't kill you then it has nothing to do with your survival instinct and your fear of it is irrational. If you don't like something or think it's wrong, that's a negative judgment and is based in irrational fear. The fear is that the thing has some power to affect your life. You want to remove the possibility of its affecting your life, so you think it would be better if that thing did not exist.

Let's take a look at something obvious: obesity. You think it is wrong for someone to be obese. You believe it's wrong because you fear it could happen to you. You might look at an extremely overweight person and judge that condition as wrong. You imagine the food they're eating or their slovenly lifestyle is responsible for their condition and you judge them as wrong. What you are really doing is creating a mental image of yourself in that condition and fearing that it could happen to you. The way you could become obese is exactly the same as the way you could become thin. You would have to be a vibrational match to it.

If you were a vibrational match to weighing four hundred pounds, you would have a very specific set of beliefs and feelings about yourself and the world around you. You would look at yourself differently in all areas of your life. You would have a certain specific set of very intense feelings about yourself. You could not weigh four hundred pounds unless you were a vibrational, emotional, and mental match to it.

The same is true of becoming a lean and healthy person. You must be a vibrational match to it. You must want it, demand it, expect it, and see yourself as it. That is the way to receive anything in this life. You must match that which you desire. The person who is fit and trim weighing one hundred and fifty pounds has a very different set of beliefs, feelings, emotions, perspective, and mental outlook than one who weighs four hundred pounds. If you want to become the lean and healthy version of yourself, you must adopt a new set of beliefs, a new perspective about life, a new persona, a new expectation of feeling good, and all of this will translate into a new vibration that matches the new version of you that you so desire.

It is not about food or how much you eat. You eat the same foods in the same amounts based on your beliefs about them and how they affect your body. When you change your beliefs, the amount and types of food you will desire will be different. The change you have made internally to your beliefs, perspective, persona, and expectations causes a change in your vibration, which causes a change in your habits. Change the inside first and the outside will match whatever vibration that comes from the change.

If you simply decide to eat differently in order to lose weight, you are trying to change the outside condition. This approach cannot work in the long term. You will always revert back to your previous state because you haven't made the necessary changes to your vibration. A lean person simply has a different vibration than a fat person. One who possesses a wonderful, loving relationship has a different set of beliefs, a different perspective, a different approach to life than one who feels lonely. Adopt the set of beliefs that allows you to receive that which you want and you will receive it.

How do you imagine a thin and healthy person thinks about food? Do they use food to soothe their uncomfortable feelings? Maybe sometimes, but probably not that often. Do they use food as entertainment? Probably not. Do they think of food as fuel? Yes, certainly. How about exercise? Do thin and healthy people sit around watching TV all day or are they constantly on the go? What do you think interests them? Activity or rest? Are they naturally this way or are they this way because their vibrations match what they want and how they see themselves?

You might look at a thin person and imagine that they were lucky for being born into their thin body. They were lucky for having thin parents and learning to eat the way thin people eat. They are naturally thin because they were born with genes that caused them to process food more efficiently. They can eat all they want because their body type burns more calories than the average person.

While it's true that everyone chose their specific body in order to create a trajectory that would lead them to what they wanted to explore in this reality, most people have a naturally lean and healthy body under all that fat. It's there waiting for them. It might not be a model's figure, but their natural shape is healthy and lean. It's just a matter of becoming a vibrational match to your own natural shape. This is accomplished by allowing for the belief that you can return to your natural shape and that your natural shape is perfect.

So what is your natural shape? If you can remember a time in your childhood when your body felt good to you, that is your natural shape. If you were lean as a child, you can become lean as an adult. If you were shapely as a child, you will be shapely as an adult. If you felt good in your body as a child, you can feel good in your adult body as well. The natural state is one that is free from stress and pressure, free from excess weight and inflammation, free from ailments, disease, aches, and pains. This is the natural state and your body can resume its perfect shape as soon as you allow it to.

Remember, you do not control your body, you influence it. Your vibration causes your body (and everything else in the universe) to match it. Change your vibration and you change your body. Match the vibration of your natural self and your body will realign itself with your ideal shape. You can't control your heart, or pancreas, or liver, or the individual cells of your body. However, your attention to unwanted things or potentially scary future conditions causes conflict and inner stress, which in turn causes stress on the body. Your body reacts by turning itself into the representation of your current vibration.

IV.

Reduce stress and you will find it easier to allow what you want to come to you, including a lean and fit body. The stress causes you to reach for outside things to soothe yourself. Imagine you are worried about money so you work extra hours hoping to relieve yourself of the worry about money. In doing so, you create stress. You eat without planning or thinking, you do not exercise, you don't get enough sleep, and you don't resolve the emotional and vibrational issues that cause you to worry in the first place. You are simply reacting to your fear by trying to change a condition that exists in your outer world. This approach does not work.

Stress is caused by an uncontrolled mind. When you imagine unpleasant future conditions, you create stress. It is fear. It is focus on what's not wanted. You can choose any thought. You can choose to imagine your future without what you want or with what you want. You can worry about this and that, but the future is an illusion. The only thing that matters is how you feel now in this present moment. Stress is caused by believing something bad will happen in the future. In order to alleviate your worries about unknown future events, you take some sort of action in the present. You are trying to move away from unwanted things rather than moving toward wanted things. This is just a habit. It is simply failing to focus on what you do want. This approach creates inner conflict and stress on the body. To soothe yourself, you react to the stress by eating without thinking. We are going to help you change your habit of thought.

Inner conflict occurs when you believe that something bad is occurring in the moment. Stress occurs when you believe that something bad will happen in the future. Relieve your inner conflict by realizing that everything is happening for you. Relieve your stress by understanding that everything is always working out for you. If you can come to this realization, you will experience far less inner conflict and stress. Why are you stressed out anyway? Let's take a closer look.

You believe that if you don't do something now, then something bad will happen in the future. We will tell you that is simply not true. You worry about having enough money to pay your bills. You worry about what others will think of you. You worry about conditions beyond your control. You worry about losing your job, your mate, or your children's love. All of this worry causes tremendous stress and pressure. It is all caused by fear. The object of your worry has no power to harm you, but ironically your worry about it is the thing that's literally killing you.

Imagine that you knew you were taken care of and that everything would always work out for you. Imagine that you could do no wrong. Imagine that it was not possible for anything to go wrong. Imagine that if something seemed to go wrong that it wasn't wrong at all, but actually it was very good indeed. It's just that from your perspective, you were unable to really see the good that would come of it. Imagine you were safe and always loved. Imagine that you could not fail. If this was the case, then you could not feel fear. If this was true, then you could not worry and without worry or negative emotion, you would not be stressed.

This is true. This is the design of physical reality. You are taken care of. Everything is working out for you. Everything is happening for you, not to you. You do create your own reality. You have the power to control your thoughts. You can free yourself of self-imposed stress and limitation. You do not need to worry, because worry does you no good. You are taken care of. That is the basis of the mechanism of physical reality. You are not alone. You really, truly have nothing to fear. Nothing bad can happen to you; it is all good and it is all for you. What you witness happening to other people is for them, not you. They are able to handle it. They have prepared themselves. Don't worry about it. Learn to see things from a higher and broader perspective.

Without the stress, worry, tension, etc., there is no need to distract or soothe yourself by reaching for things in your outer world. By thinking clearly about what you do want rather than worrying about what you do not want, you relieve stress and turn your power of attention on the creation of whatever it is that you prefer. By not trying to control others so that you can feel better, you allow them to be who they are while maintaining your focus on their positive aspects.

V.

The realization that you are taken care of, that everything is happening for you, and that everything is always working out for you will give you ease. Ease creates an environment of allowing. In this environment, where you have little stress, where you understand that there is nothing to worry about, where you are able to know the purpose of your emotions, where you are not trying to change the conditions in the moment, where you are focused on what it is you really want, you become an allower. Everything you want flows to you in this state. In the allowing state there is little resistance. Whenever a little resistance shows itself by way of some negative emotion, you react by going inside, finding the fear, and practicing the art of analysis.

This approach to life is fully aligned with the laws of the universe as we know them. Allow what you want to come to you and drop your resistance to what is. See that your perspective is limited and reach for the higher perspective. Believe that what we have told you is true and you will begin a new life from this moment forward. Know that you have nothing to fear in your emotions. They are for your guidance. There is nothing wrong with negative emotions and they are to be cherished, not feared. When you feel negative emotion, you will now realize that there is some limiting belief to uncover and that belief is based in irrational fear. That's all the emotion is telling you. There's nothing more to it than that. You are not bad or wrong for anything. You are just looking at yourself, or others, or the event, from a limited perspective that is not true.

Living a life of ease is your birthright. Living a life of struggle is unnecessary. Your struggle (or resistance) has caused you to gain weight. Your struggle has created a habit of fear and worry. Your struggle has caused you to be fearful. By demanding to feel good, you can now deal with that irrational fear and return to a life of ease. You no longer need to prove your worthiness. You no longer need to pretend to be someone you're not. You can be yourself and know that your unique perspective on life proves that you are a worthy being.

Now it is time to control your mind. Now it is time to free your mind. Now it is time to demand that you feel good. Now it is finally time to think of yourself. This is your universe and everything revolves around you. You must begin to start thinking in a way that empowers you. You must begin to think fearlessly. You must pay a little more attention to the thoughts you chronically think. You must work to free yourself of your limiting beliefs. This is the only thing you need to do. Nothing else really matters. When you begin to place how you feel above all else, everything else will magically move into place.

Your body will respond when you feel good. When you feel good you will relieve your body of the stress and inner conflict that has accumulated over time. Your body will allow well-being to flow once again. Your body will begin to take its natural shape. Your body will urge you not to reach for a quick fix because you won't need anything outside yourself. Instead, your body will guide you to what it needs to fuel itself and to create optimum health and well-being. This is the system that was designed for you. You will thrive when you release your self-imposed stress. Do whatever it takes to feel good. Place feeling good above all else and you will see the results you desire. Not only will your body return to its optimum weight and health, but all areas of your life will improve as well.

Your relationships will become better and stronger. You will experience more abundance than ever before. You will be guided toward your passions and interests. You will move toward the state of bliss. You will grow spiritually. You will move rapidly toward being who you really are. You will contribute to the elevation of the planet's consciousness. When you make your world better, you make the whole world better. You are the center of your universe. It's now time to define your universe using the knowledge and power you hold within yourself. It is time for you to take control.

You are loved more than you could imagine by more than you could ever count.

We Are Joshua

Chapter Sixteen

What To Do Next

We understand that this is not a typical diet book. We also realize that you would prefer to be told what to do. To you it may seem easier to follow a set of instructions and complete a set of tasks. Unfortunately, this cannot work. There are no instructions to follow, nor any tasks to complete. If we gave you some things to do that would lead to weight loss, the results would be the same as all the other diets. Nothing can work for you unless it resonates with your vibration and only when you have altered your vibration to become a match to the lean body you desire. So then we ask you one thing: are you a match to the lean body you desire? Are you on your way to becoming a match? Are you in the process of altering your limiting beliefs? Are you becoming an allower? If so, that is very good indeed and we will suggest some things you might want to try if you are inspired to do so.

1. Meditation

First of all we ask that you begin to practice meditation. Daily meditation will help you to take control over the thoughts you think. It is a mental practice that works to exercise the most powerful aspect of your human existence. You must learn to have some control over the thoughts you think. Meditation helps you in this area. Until you can consciously control your thoughts, you will continue to receive a mix of beneficial and limiting thoughts. In order to reach the vibration that matches what you want, you must exercise some form of control over your thoughts.

Time spent meditating daily is time well spent. In your quest to sculpt your body into the shape you prefer, you will want to do certain things. Nothing is more beneficial than fifteen to twenty minutes of meditation each day. We have created a series of meditations that you can use to get started in your practice. Each meditation covers a different topic that will raise your vibration and help you get into alignment with the things you desire most. These topics are health and well-being, money and abundance, relationships and love, spirituality, worthiness, and appreciation and gratitude.

In the beginning it will take some patience to become accustomed to this new form of exercise. Like any exercise, it may feel uncomfortable in the beginning. However, after a few days you will pick up on the cadence and rhythm of the meditation and you will learn to relax your mind and slow down thought. With further practice you will be able to stop thought altogether for a few moments and then the duration of thought-free periods will increase. Soon you will have awareness and control of your thoughts.

Meditation will help you open the channel between you and your inner self. Your inner self is fully aware of you and every thought you think. Your inner self is always connected to you and lives life with you in every moment. There is never a time that your inner self is not fully present with you in your body. However, you are relatively unaware of the presence of your inner self. Meditation will help you regain awareness of your inner self.

When you regain your awareness of the presence of your inner self, you can start a dialogue. You can begin to receive communication from your inner self. You will begin to hear the words, think the thoughts, and receive the inspiration that is being given to you by your inner self. This is a heightened level of physical existence. Inspiration to act at this level of understanding and consciousness comes from a much higher and broader perspective. It engages and leverages the forces of the universe.

The highest form of physical existence is the blending of one with their inner self. Living as your inner self while on Earth fully engages and utilizes universal forces and the higher perspective in every moment. Meditation will allow you to move toward this state of being.

Daily meditation using a guide will help you unlock your limitations in certain areas. If you feel unworthy, as most do, you might benefit from the guided meditation on worthiness. Hearing that you are worthy helps you feel worthy and as you feel more worthy, your vibration is raised and your reality takes shape to reflect that new vibration. As long as you believe what you hear, your world will alter itself to reflect your newer, higher beliefs.

Meditation has the effect of altering your reality because it allows you to take control of your thoughts. When you begin to consciously choose more empowering thoughts, you raise your vibration. Higher vibrations lead to improved experiences. You came here to explore reality without limitations. The way to do that is by removing your self-imposed limitations and meditation is an excellent way to start.

2. Appreciation

Getting to wherever you want to go is through the path of appreciating what you have now. It may seem counter-intuitive. You may think that where you want to be is so much better than where you are now. You may even hate certain aspects of your current life. However, hating something, disliking something, being in resistance to something that exists now, keeps your focus of attention squarely on the thing you do not like. When you notice the negative aspects of something, what you are actually doing is asking the universe to bring you more of that.

By loving the positive aspects of anything, including your body and even the fat cells in your body, you are not asking the universe to bring you more fat, you are asking the universe to bring you more love. When you notice that your hair is shiny, or your eyes are blue, or your teeth are free of cavities, or you appreciate your smile, or anything about yourself at all, you are expressing love. You are looking at yourself in a loving way and the universe will bring you more things to love. That's just how the system works.

When you dislike something, you are expressing fear. "What if I can't lose weight? What will people think of me? No one will like me. My mate will leave me." It's not that you don't appreciate your body, it's that your body is causing you to feel fear. There's nothing wrong with your body as it is right now. In a natural world, free from fear and stress, you would not care about the shape of your body. By not caring, it would take its natural shape. It's only because you think that a fat body means something that you care. You look at your body and your imagination races. You feel fear because you have not yet learned to control the thoughts you think. If you could control your thoughts, you would not feel fear; you would appreciate the body as it is and your body would allow well-being to flow. The body would take its natural shape.

Appreciation will help you accept your body as it is and reduce the fear associated with your current perspective. There is nothing inherently wrong with a body that is a few pounds over its normal weight. In fact, we know that in many cases a few extra pounds is healthy. It's your perspective that makes you think that you and your body are wrong for being overweight. If you had a different perspective, you would feel differently about your body. There would be no fear.

What if you thought it was attractive to be fat? What if you believed that others thought highly of you because of your shapely figure? What if it was a sign of wealth? Just a few decades ago, many people thought it was fashionable to be a few pounds heavier than the rest. It showed status. People enjoyed being overweight. It made them feel good. They liked everything about it, including the food. They saw no reason to think harshly about themselves.

Your weight is a matter of perspective. To some you are fat and no matter how much weight you lose, you will always be fat to them. To others you are the perfect weight and they wish they looked as good as you. You can't maintain a weight that will appeal to all people, so there's no point in trying. Don't worry what others think, because it has nothing to do with you. From their perspective you are probably either too fat or too thin.

All you can consider is how you feel in your body. If being leaner feels good, then that can lead to the lean body you desire. If your present weight feels good, then that's perfect. If you enjoy all the things that come with the few extra pounds you carry with you, then you can live a very happy and healthy life. It only matters what you think and there is no wrong way to think. Do whatever feels good to you, but leave everyone else out of it.

You will learn what feels good to you by being honest with yourself. You must consider that most aspects of your physical body are excellent and you would not trade them for anyone else's. Take each individual piece of your physical body and think about how wonderful it is. Your feet are excellent at walking. You can paint your toenails. Your shins are perfectly shaped. You knees bend easily. You arms are smooth. Your heart beats easily without you having to do anything. You can look at any individual piece of your body and you can claim it as perfect and wonderful or you can despise it as hideous and gross. It is all up to you.

You are in control of this exercise. You can choose to see the positive aspects of every single part of your body or you can choose to find fault. You must be honest and make the choice. If you are going to be determined to keep finding fault, then you are cementing your own fate. You will continue to struggle through life complaining about what is and noticing that things never change. Or you can begin to appreciate the same things you dislike. You can start looking at the positives and release your grasp on the negative. Nothing is inherently good or bad; it is all neutral. It is your personal judgment that causes something to be right or wrong. You can choose to see how everything is right, good, and positive. It's a matter of choice and perspective.

Believe us when we tell you that appreciation is the fastest way to get anything you want. By loving what is, you bring more love into your life. Appreciation causes love to grow. It causes good to get better. It causes right to become even more right for you. It makes the positive aspects seem even more positive. Appreciation is the most powerful tool of creation. You got everything you ever received because you appreciated it before you got it.

It is more effective when you physically write in a journal a list of things you appreciate on a daily basis. Write down things you appreciate about your body as it is now, but don't stop there. Continue writing about everything you appreciate. Realize that it was you, through the alignment and focus of your vibration, that allowed everything you appreciate to become part of your reality. You created everything you have in your life and the vast majority of it is very good indeed. Write a daily list, in your own hand with pen and paper, of at least five things you appreciate. Do this for thirteen weeks in a row without missing one day and by the end of the time period you will have altered your perspective to such a degree that your life will be forever changed for the better.

3. Gratitude

Appreciation helps you bring into focus the things in your life that you like. From a stance of appreciation, you give yourself credit and feel proud of creating and attracting those things you like that exist in your life now.

Gratitude, by comparison, gives thanks for the system that allows you to create that which you desire. Gratitude gives thanks to the universe, to your idea of God, to the mechanism of physical reality, to your inner self, to your guides, and to all the entities within All That Is who help you to create the life you desire.

When you appreciate your body, you can feel proud for the creation that is your body. You created your body, as well as all of the parts and pieces that make up your body. You coordinated the design and creation of that which is your body through your intentions prior to your emergence into this physical reality. You created the relationships you enjoy, the work you do now, the home you live in, as well as everything else and you should feel good for what you have created. It is truly magnificent.

There is another side to the creation of your life that you might not consider to be your creation, but you are thankful that it is there. While you might appreciate your mate, you might give gratitude to the Law of Attraction for bringing you together. You might give thanks to him for loving you as he does. You might be thankful to her for allowing you to see your fears and limiting beliefs. You might give thanks to yourself for allowing yourself to receive that which you desire.

Gratitude and appreciation go hand in hand. You appreciate what you know that you've created and you give thanks to all that assists you in the creation process. You might be thankful for the universe for leading you to this book, or to another teacher, or for your ability to recognize that which resonates in a deeper part of your being.

When you give thanks for things that have not yet shown up in your reality, you practice the art of faith. This is a very powerful act of creation. When you thank yourself for having faith that you can create the lean body you desire and for those who will guide you to the proper foods, the proper instruction, the proper exercise, the proper approach to sculpting the body you prefer, the aligned mindset, and all the beneficial beliefs you will need, you are displaying your faith in those who are there to guide you toward that which will enable you to engage the forces of the universe and move effortlessly in the direction you prefer. You are not in this alone. By expressing gratitude, you include all of those who are there supporting you, encouraging you, and guiding you. This is the leverage you need to get whatever it is that you desire.

Just as you will engage the power of appreciation through daily journal writing, so will you engage the power of gratitude. In the same journal, write a list of at least five things you can be thankful for each and every day. Think of your guides and your inner self. Imagine that they are fully aware of you and know how to get you where you want to go. Remember that your perspective is limited, but their perspective is not. They can see things you can't see. They know things you can't know. They understand to a higher degree how the universe works. Give thanks to them for guiding you. Give thanks to the mechanism of physical reality for allowing you to experience life in such grand detail. Give thanks every day and you will notice a significant shift in the quality of your daily experience of life.

4. Intention

There is no greater tool for creating what you want in the moment than intention. This is a powerful tool that you may not have been aware of previously. When you intend for something to happen, you are pre-paving your own future. You are choosing a perspective in advance. You are focusing your powers of creation. You are choosing, in advance, what you prefer.

You may set your intentions before you begin your day. You might intend to enjoy a nice breakfast with your mate. You might intend to have a smooth and uneventful commute to work. You might intend to be productive, have fun, be aware, and look for positive aspects throughout your day. You might intend to go out with friends for a nice dinner. You might intend to read something fun before bed. And before going to sleep, you can intend to sleep well, have pleasant dreams, be well rested, and of course wake up the next morning.

You may set your intentions before every event. When walking into a meeting, set your intentions for what you want to happen. Before making a phone call, set your intentions for what you would like to communicate. Before writing an email, set your intentions to write clearly and for the other person to understand your words and tone. When you set your intentions, you engage the powers of the universe to create something more effective.

You want to sculpt a lean and healthy body. Food, water, exercise, rest, and ease will help you create the body you desire. Before ordering or preparing a meal, intend for it to be healthy, flavorful, satisfying, and contributing to your overall health and well-being. Before you eat, intend for the food to be distributed throughout your body in order to feed the cells and deliver the nutrients to wherever they are required. Imagine that your body is a system, a community, and that you are providing the community with all it needs to live happily and to continue thriving.

If you would simply set your intentions at the beginning of every day, writing down what you intended to eat, what you intended to do for exercise, how much water you intended to drink, and an intention to be mindful and pay attention to conflict and stress, you would intentionally create the lean body of your dreams.

5. Affirmations

You are not a vibrational match to the lean body you desire. You have some beliefs that hold you apart from whatever it is that you want. In order to become a vibrational match to anything wanted, you must alter your vibration. The way to do that is by thinking a bit differently than you do now. Part of that is accomplished by thinking differently about yourself. You have certain limiting beliefs that are not true and by reminding yourself of your absolute worthiness, you can alter the intensity of those beliefs.

We suggest the following affirmations that are absolutely true for you because they are true for everyone. You must not only speak affirmations to yourself, but you must write them in your own hand on paper every single day. The daily practice of writing down affirmations will cause the shift that will begin to alter your reality.

I am a worthy being.

I am worthy of everything I desire.

I am unique to all the universe.

No one like me has ever lived before or will ever live again.

I create my own reality through the thoughts I think.

I can choose to think any thought I like.

I have free will.

I can decide to judge things as good or bad. That is my choice.

I can choose to see the good in everything because I am good.

I am a unique expression of Source, God, All That Is and therefore I am worthy.

I exist, therefore I am. I am eternal.

I cannot fail, because there is only expansion, there is never failure.

I have a right to enjoy my life the way I deem it to be. I can choose anything. It is up to me.

This is my universe. Everything in my universe is happening for me.

I am being flooded with well-being. I can choose to allow the well-being to flow or I can choose to limit that flow anytime I want.

I am good.

I am wonderful as I am.

I am perfect in this moment as I am and I improve with each new moment.

I am strong.

Everything is always working out for me.

I have the divine right to have, be, and do anything.

I am a limitless being of unconditional love and acceptance.

I can choose anything.

I can choose to be right or I can choose not to. It is all up to me.

I can create ease in my life. I have total control over every aspect of my life.

I understand that sometimes I choose to look at things from the limited perspective, but I have the ability to choose to see things from the higher perspective if I want to.

I feel good. I can choose to feel good.

I appreciate how good it is to feel good and I choose to feel good.

This is a feeling reality and the only thing that really matters is how I feel and therefore I choose to feel good as much of the time as possible.

I explore contrast in order to define my preferences.

I do not make mistakes, I choose to explore contrast.

I am an explorer and I choose to explore reality in my own unique way. Therefore, I know I cannot do wrong, be wrong, or get it wrong.

I am right.

There is no wrong anywhere in the universe; that is the proof that I am right.

Everyone else is right too.

From their perspective, in their universe, they are being right for them and

I can respect that.

I do not have to follow unless I want to follow. I do not have to lead unless I choose to lead. It is all up to me.

I enjoy my life.

I enjoy the feeling of anticipation, surprise, wonder, and curiosity.

I am a freedom seeking being and I choose to recognize the freedom I have to create whatever I want.

There is no bad or wrong, only judgments that create the illusion of bad or wrong.

I am free.

I am alive.

I have physical senses that allow me to enjoy and explore physical reality. I have nonphysical senses that allow me to perceive the reality of my reality.

I am loved.

I am love.

I am supported by the universe.

I am supported by my inner self.

I am supported by many nonphysical guides.

I am fully supported in every single moment by countless physical and nonphysical entities.

I have the power of the universe supporting me in every moment.

I am right, good, and perfect as I am.

I am the authentic representation of a truly unique point of view.

I am valuable.

I am a valuable part of the universe.

Without me, the universe would be less than it is.

I am required.

I am necessary.

I am needed, but I do not need anything.

I am self-contained.

I have unique talents and abilities.

I am a unique representation of Source.

I am an eternal being living a physical existence in order to explore reality and expand in joy.

I seek joy.

I am joy.

I love joy and joy is a representation of who I really am.

I am ease.

I am calm.

I enjoy the variety of my emotions and I wonder at the depth and complexity of feeling.

I appreciate my inner guidance system that proves I am supported.

The list of possible affirmations is endless. Write at least five affirmations every day with pen and paper and your limiting beliefs will begin to fade away into oblivion.

6. The Playbook

As you may have already noticed by now, The Joshua Diet is not really a diet at all. It is an approach to life. The goal is not to lose weight, to become more healthy, or to become rich, successful, or even create wonderful relationships. The goal is to become an allower and then simply allow everything you want to flow to you. By replacing struggle with ease, you create an environment of allowing. By making life fun rather than hard work, you engage the forces of the universe. Everything you have been told up to this point in time has been the old approach to life. The new approach is far more effective, more joyful, more rewarding, and a whole lot more fun. The new approach will be a life where you feel very good most of the time. In those rare moments when you feel bad, you will notice it and you will seek to understand the message behind the manifestation event.

The side effect of living in this new way will be the lean body you prefer, the best health you could imagine, the most loving relationships you could conceive, the success and abundance you desire, and the ease you've always wanted. The universe knows what you want. You've been asking for it your whole life. It's been on its way to you since the first day you asked for it, but you've been unconsciously resisting it. This new approach is a way of life where you consciously allow it all to flow to you.

It is not goal-oriented, it is feeling-oriented. It is an intentional way of living. It is a conscious way of life. It is an awakened method of moving through the experience of physical reality. You are aware that this is all for you. You are aware that you have complete control over the creation of your experience. You are aware that others cannot create in your reality. You allow everything to unfold as it will because this is the path of least resistance. The less resistance you have to life, the more of what you want will come to you.

This is a book of ideas and information. Depending on your current state of being, you have been able to absorb much (but not all) of the information contained in this book. We have not told you what to eat, how to exercise, what to avoid, or any specific steps you need to take to physically lose the weight you desire. That is because you are unique. No one program can work for everyone. In fact, most programs cannot work for most people in the long term. Until you adjust your view of life, you cannot make any long-term lasting changes. First you change your approach to life, then you will be inspired to find the program that works for you.

When you change your approach to life, your vibration will change. This sends a new signal out to the universe and it responds by creating a reality that matches your new, higher vibration. You will be inspired to read articles, visit websites, watch TV shows, overhear conversations, meet new people, and many other things. Each will lead you down a path to discovering that which will align with your unique body. You might be inspired to try a new cuisine, to try a new sport, to become interested in cooking, to become a vegetarian, or to modify your diet in some other way. Nothing will seem like work. It will all be fun and interesting. You will feel alive. You will not feel struggle, effort, or dissatisfaction.

If something comes along and it is not fun or particularly interesting, it is not for you. If it doesn't feel good, it's not for you. If it's a struggle, it's not for you. It will be fun, it will be interesting, and you will find it easy. If it doesn't meet this criteria, it's not for you and you can leave it alone.

If you're receiving inspiration, you have reached a new vibrational level and you've incorporated what you have read in this book. If you are not receiving inspiration, you are still in a state of resistance. Ease your fears, ease your resistance, and begin allowing. Reread this book over and over again. We know it is repetitive. It is meant to be repetitive. You are meant to "get it" at some point. You have been living a resistant life for a long time and the thought of ease is foreign to you. Ease is the way. Struggle just does not work. You must understand this point before anything can change.

Understanding what we are saying intellectually is all well and good. Now you need to put it into practice. Now you must incorporate it into the fabric of your life. We ask that you spend a few minutes everyday intentionally creating your life. You do a lot of things every single day that keep the train going down the same old tracks. Now it's time to switch tracks. Now it's time to take a little time to intentionally create the life you prefer. Reading about it is one thing; taking action is something that will incorporate what you have learned into your life. It is this action that will create the life you desire. A few minutes each day will cause the shift you are looking for.

We have created The Joshua Diet Playbook. This playbook is designed to focus your attention on the positive aspects of all areas of your life. There are exercises that will promote a set of highly beneficial beliefs and cause you to bring your attention to what is wanted, rather than what is unwanted. The exercises must be completed in the evening prior to the next day or in the morning of each day. The workbook lasts for thirteen weeks and that first book will create a great shift in your life. But we ask that you do not stop and rather keep going and continue practicing every single day for an entire year. And when the year is up and your life is brighter, continue for another year and another year after that and so on and so on.

You are where you are due to the thoughts you've been thinking your entire life. Now it's time to bring in some new and more powerful thoughts. You've arrived at this place in your life and that is very good. Everything has unfolded perfectly to bring you here. Your vibration has never been higher. This is a crucial point in your life. You must move forward or you will revert to the same old thoughts and beliefs that created all of what you do not want. Let's change those thoughts. Let's incorporate new beliefs. Let's take control of your life and actively create the life you prefer. You can do it, but you must practice.

Start today and commit to a life-long practice of focus and intention. Become who you want to be by learning to shape your beliefs about yourself. Whether you believe it or not, you create your own reality. Whether you believe it or not, you are worthy. Whether you believe it or not, you are unique. Whether you believe it or not, you can have, be, and do anything you want. You have taken the first step by reading this book, but there is more to it than that. You must put what you've learned into action. You must recognize that there is more to do. You must make use of aids that are available to you. You must carve out a few minutes each day to actively shape your perception of reality.

The Joshua Diet Playbook will not help you if you haven't read The Joshua Diet and the Joshua Diet will be far less effective if you don't use the Joshua Playbook everyday. The Playbook is a very powerful tool. Your commitment to completing the daily exercises is an empowering decision. Your vibration will rise every day. You will undergo a change. You will become a newer, higher version of yourself. You will start to notice your reality shifting.

In a short time you will begin to see signs in your reality that are a match to your higher vibration. Things will get better. Life will become easier. Your resistance will fade and your struggle will start to be replaced with ease. When you practice these exercises every morning or every evening, you will begin to feel differently about yourself, your life, and those around you. You will notice that your clothes fit better. You will notice that people are responding to you differently. You will observe that things are starting to work out for you more often. You will begin to feel much better.

You may not lose ten pounds in three weeks, but gradually, you will see signs that things are shifting. You might not come into a fortune overnight, but you will notice little signs of abundance all around you. You might not meet the mate of your dreams in the first month, but you will notice more people smiling at you, you will feel more attractive, and you will be more open to meeting new people. Everything will become a little clearer and brighter. Everything will get better.

By practicing your powers of creation a little every day, your life will begin to unfold in ways you cannot imagine. If you will simply do the exercises every single day, without missing too many days, without considering it work, without complaining that it takes too much time, without worrying that you're missing out on something else, the quality of your life experience will radically improve. A year from now, you will look back to where you are now and you will not be able to believe that you traveled so far in such a short amount of time.

You cannot imagine the version of you that will exist one year from now. You would not recognize yourself. You will be different. Every thought you are thinking now will be replaced with higher-vibrational thoughts.

All of your limiting beliefs will be diminished so much that you will not recognize them. You will think of yourself differently. You will no longer be defensive. You will no longer suffer through hurt feelings. You will have great confidence. You will feel more love and joy in your life. You will be inspired to do so many more things. You will have less fear. You will be fitter and healthier than you could conceive. You will enjoy life.

If you take time to practice the creation of you, we promise that you will appreciate what you've created. We can see the real you. We know what you can become. We see your potential. We know far more than we can tell you in this short book. There's only one thing you have to do: have faith that we know what we are talking about. Have faith that there is a life for you beyond your wildest imagination and that you can get there. Have faith that you will enjoy this process of transformation. Have faith that everything is working out for you. Have faith that an easing of resistance will allow you to create the life of your dreams. Have faith that you have the power to create your own reality. Have faith that all is well. Have faith that it will work for you. Have faith that you cannot fail. Have faith that things will get better. Have faith that it's all in your hands.

It's all up to you. It's all in your power. The next few days are crucial. Decide what you want to do next. Release the fear and choose to move toward that which you have always wanted. Make a commitment now. Do it for you, for your loved ones and for the shared consciousness of the planet. Make the decision now. Write it down. What are you going to do?

I AM _____

_____

_____

_____

_____

_____

_____

_____

Testimonials

I wanted to thank you from the bottom of my heart, for bringing Joshua's answer to me.

When I read the message, I burst into tears, because of joy and relief. And I couldn't think of anything but "Thank you, thank you, thank you... Thank you Gary, thank you Joshua, thank you my God." Now I keep reading the answer with the intention to absorb the message. Love ~**Marine**

Thank you so very much for answering my question. Having read Joshua's answer three times so far, I'm already feeling better, more confident and exited about the future. ~**Alette**

Many thanks for such a prompt reply. It makes so much sense and I have to say that reading Joshua's response I have had the biggest shift/insight/aha moment ever.

So thank you, thank you, thank you. How empowering, how amazing!!! ~**Fabienne**

Much love and appreciation to you, Gary, and to Joshua for your prompt and most enlightening response to my question. ~**Debra**

What a beautiful relaxing answer. Source provides everything — my responsibility is to allow it and yes, I see how my belief system, with some helpful beliefs and a lot of limiting beliefs, keeps me where I am. ~**Kate**

Wow, it's wonderful, powerful answer and I really get it. It makes me feel so much better! I'm also happy to realize that what I've done with her has been the 'right' thing to do. I've discussed my feelings about it with a friend and my husband but I haven't talked to her about it other than to just casually ask her something about it a couple of times. Each time she had nothing really to say about things and I never pushed it. I had decided early on to basically follow her lead on things regarding the friends. I'm relieved to know that I have handled that 'right' and most likely haven't changed her trajectory. I am so thankful to have this source, both you and Joshua. ~**Tasha**

You do great work Gary. Thank you so much for all you do to help us live with a greater understanding of how reality works down here so we can have more joy and happiness. ~**Cass**

Gary, I just finished listening to your show tonight and it was amazing. I think this one was my favourite. I have to say that all of you are so down to earth and fun that I feel like I know you all. Steve always says exactly what I feel! What he said tonight about just about making a breakthrough with himself hit it on the nail for me. ~**Pamela**

Woah, this is a HUGE answer. Yet more proof I need to work on my insecurities or being judged. Just like the lady on the airplane in the summer ;-) as well as to quit looking for imperfections in others; to empathize that their life experience has been vastly different to mine. Therefore if they act out of fear, that's okay. I can hold my head above the water or let the negative vibe pull me down. It's only a choice of focus and alignment.

Thank you so much once again. I am going to read this a few times more! ~**Sam**

I am loving all the Joshua synchronicities today. Thank you so much for the 10 life ideas from Joshua. I have printed them out to help me on my never ending search for life's meanings. Much Love ~**Denise**

Thank you so much for your quick reply of Joshua's answer. Do I need to tell you that I cried while reading Joshua's answer? :-) ~**Audrey**

Thank you for such elevating wisdom. What a difference it makes to my perspective!!

Alexander loves super heroes more than anything. I will reframe the story and he will love it. ~**Lis**

Thank you so very much for sharing the new book with me!! I have come a long way since my first question, just focusing on Joshua's words daily has allowed me to move my vibration slowly in the right direction. I do know I am powerful ~ and when I keep my focus on their teachings, I see TREMENDOUS improvements in my health. I am also learning when I focus on the negative, I fall right back into the hole. This answer ~ and their reference to acceptance ~ resonates with my very soul ~ so thank you again for bringing this to me! I am enjoying your radio show ~ I look forward to it each week!! Thank you for offering it to us all!! **~Wendy**

Many thanks to Joshua, and to you, Gary, for allowing them to work through you. I felt love in the response, and the speed with which it was delivered. I received your email at the perfect moment this morning, as I was rushing off to work, and it set the perfect tone for my day. I look forward to reading it many more times. ~Kyla

Thanks so much Gary (and Joshua). As usual your answer is invaluable. Much gratitude and love. ~Jacky

I just loved Joshua's answer. It actually made me cry and I was so excited to read it. It was really really amazing and smart!! Every word of it. I will probably read it again tomorrow and the day after, and the next day and the next..... **~Shira**

Thank you so much for Joshua's answer which has given me much to ponder over and reflect on. He has (sic: they have) made me more conscious of the parts of me that sometimes appear which are not truly in alignment with who I really am. The brilliant news is that I do recognize them and now I can go about doing something about them, They are exactly caused through fear. Fear of not being good enough — I am a perfectionist — well actually I am a recovering perfectionist!! **~Jean**

I was one of those people who thought she knew quite a lot about how the Universe works, and how we work within it. And although I did know about each section in this book, I found I was missing a link, a vital key, how it all fits together to actually WORK! Gary's channel to Joshua is incredibly clear. I have learnt so much in this book that I feel I have gone through a massive internal shift and transformation taking me higher than I have ever been before on the journey of my Soul. This is a book that should be taught at school....OH if only! One day perhaps. ~**Kirsten**

If you would like to read questions from people all over the world and Joshua's answers, please visit

www.theteachingsofjoshua.com

16154606R00128

Printed in Poland
by Amazon Fulfillment
Poland Sp. z o.o., Wrocław